2004

Mommy,

I thought you would want this back.

Lots of love,

Phoebe

XO XO XO XO XO XO XO XO XO XOXO

Heaven Scent

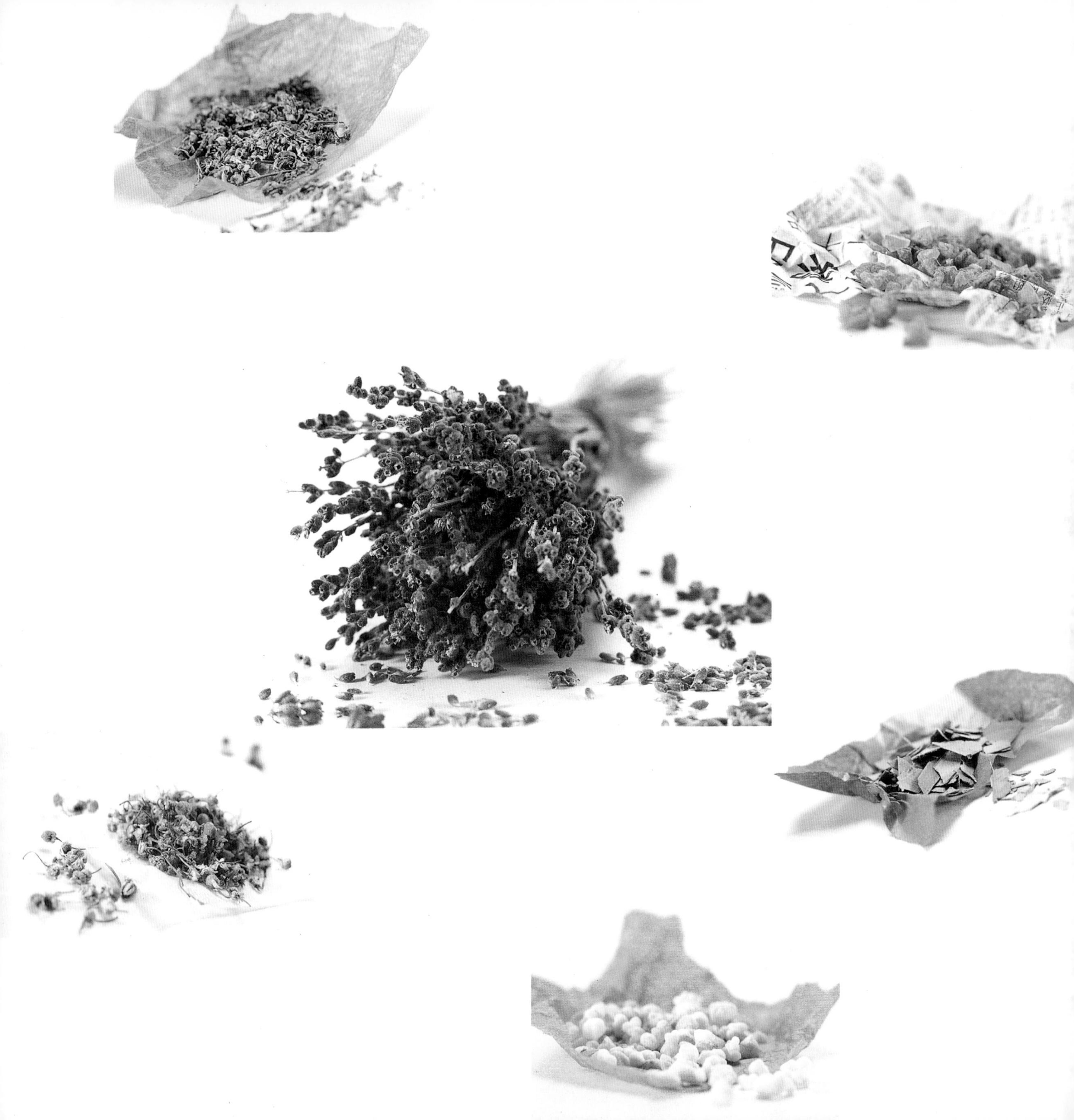

Heaven Scent

Aromatic Gifts to Make, Send, and Keep

Labeena Ishaque

Watson-Guptill Publications
New York

First published in the United States in 1998 by
Watson-Guptill Publications, a division of
BPI Communications, Inc., 1515 Broadway, New York,
NY 10036

Library of Congress Cataloging-in-Publication Data
Ishaque, Labeena.
Heaven scent: aromatic gifts to make, send, and keep/Labeena Ishaque
p. cm.
ISBN 0-8230-2238-2 (cloth)
1. Handicraft. 2. Potpourris (Scented floral mixtures) 3. Gifts.
I. Title.
TT157.I76. 1998
745.5—dc21 98-24729
CIP

This book was designed and produced by
Quintet Publishing Limited
The Old Brewery
6 Blundell Street
London N7 9BH

CREATIVE DIRECTOR: **richard dewing**
ART DIRECTOR: **silke braun**
DESIGN: **balley design associates**
DESIGNERS: **simon balley and joanna hill**
SENIOR EDITOR: **laura sandelson**
EDITOR: **lyn coutts**
PHOTOGRAPHER: **tim ferguson hill**

Printed in Singapore

First printing, 1998

contents

chapter 1

perfume through the ages 6

chapter 2

the perfume directory 20

chapter 3

essential oils and aromatherapy 36

chapter 4

scent with love 52

chapter 5

fragrant pampering 82

chapter 6

the aromatic home 110

templates 138

index 144

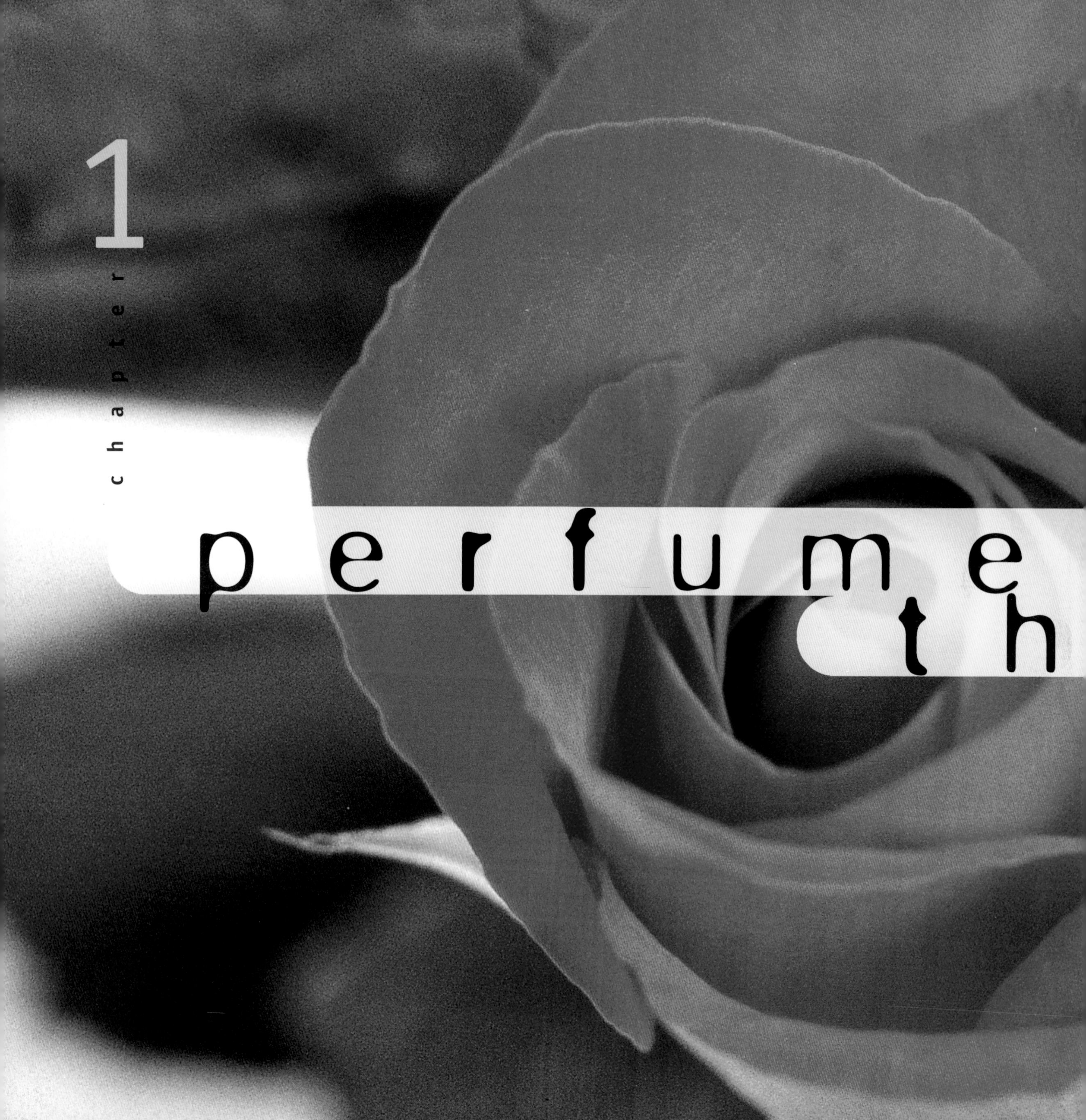
1
chapter
perfume
th

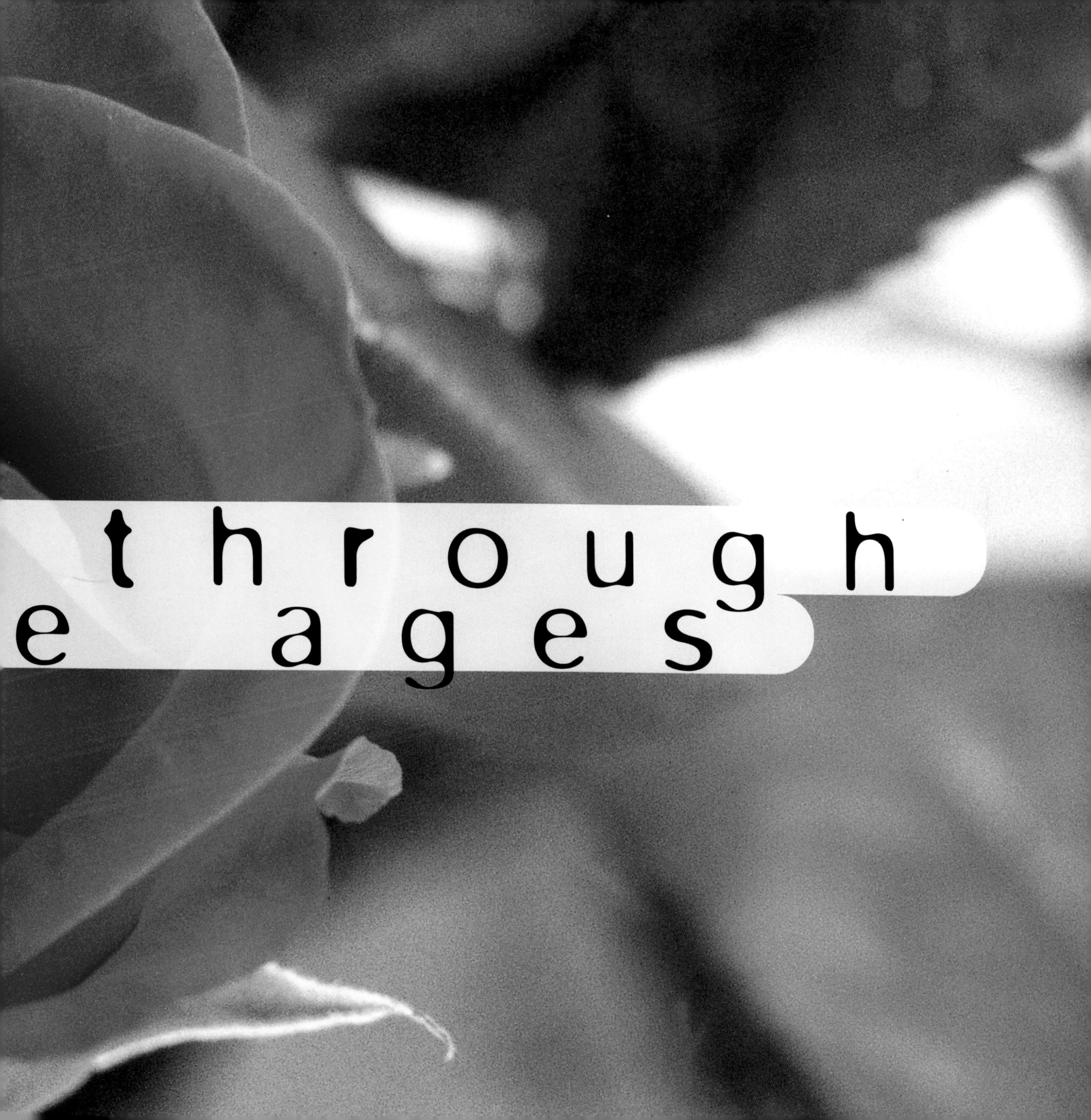
through
e ages

PERFUMES IN ANTIQUITY

Since the beginning of history humankind has associated scent with some curious and somewhat contradictory ideals. On one hand it has been associated with good health, science, and religion. On the other, scent was all about indulgence, illusion, magic, and secularity. These opposing notions though go a long way toward explaining just how complex and sensitive is our sense of smell. It also highlights the latent power of perfume and its almost mystical appeal. Perfume creates illusions that vary with the fragrance and with the wearer's or passer-by's preconception or expectation of that fragrance. Whether plant scents evoke in you a sense of well-being and cleanliness, or aromatic spices resonate with things spiritual, perfume has a story to tell.

Before we follow the story of perfume by looking at its history, let's first become familiar with our sense of smell.

our most powerful sense

The reason that one smell may attract while another repels is because the sensors in our nose are connected to the olfactory nerve. When the olfactory nerve reacts to a fragrance it affects a part of the brain called the limbic system that controls our emotions, sex drive, and thus our motivations. How these three react determines our response to a fragrance.

But it's not quite as straightforward as that because a perfume—or indeed any odor—can contain many different fragrances. Therefore our response to a perfume depends on which fragrance or fragrances the limbic system locks onto, and this can change as often as our emotions or indeed our sex drive! The combinations of fragrances in just one perfume can be so numerous that a room full of people may well have totally different reactions to it. But now for the goods news—the human nose is so sensitive that it can detect a scent that is present in only a most minute quantity. Even better, a smell can be

below: ***The Sense of Smell*** **by the French artist Arnoult.**

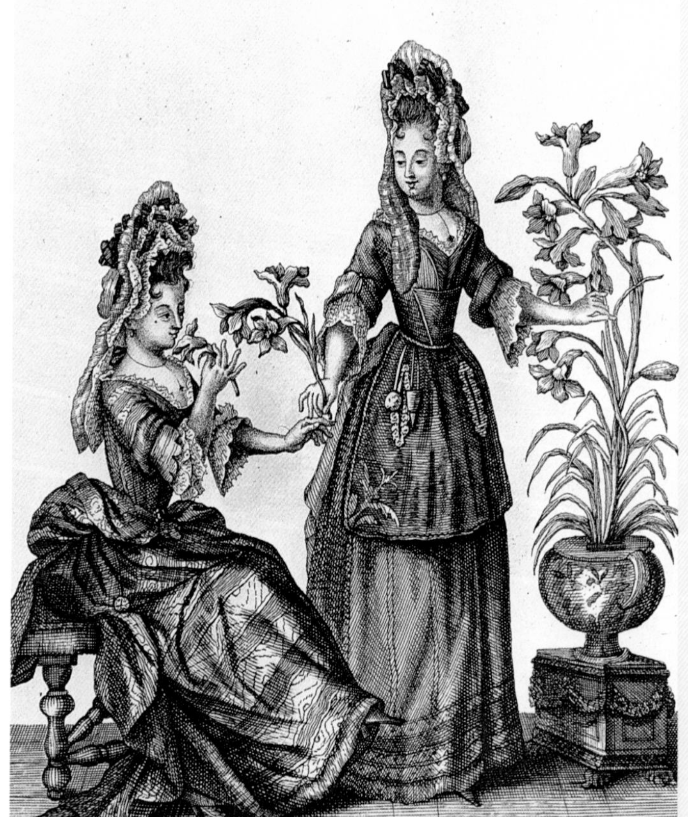

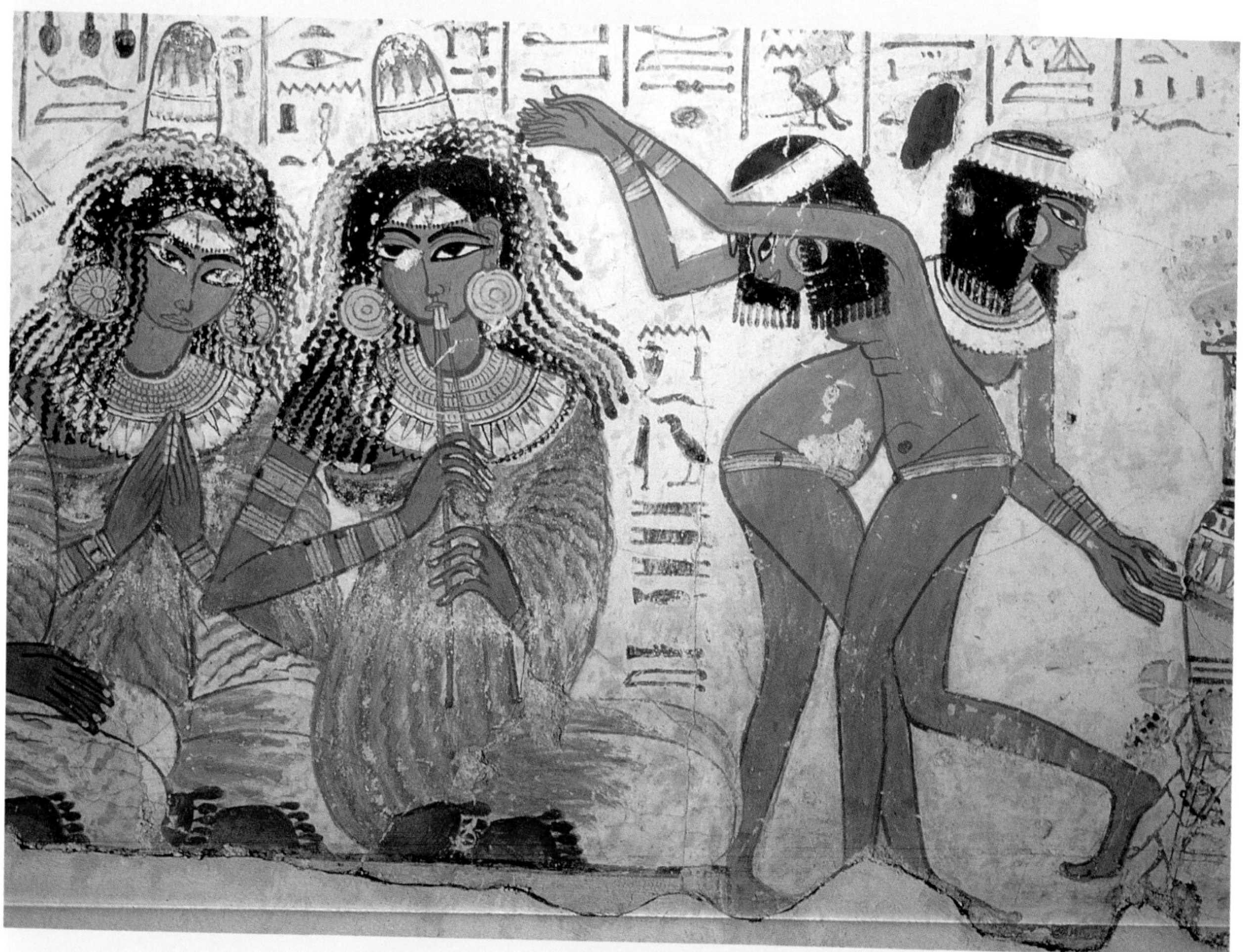

recalled or its association rekindled long after you think you've forgotten it. For example, you may be standing next to someone on a bus and if their smell is attractive and recalled, you will automatically turn to look at them. But before your eyes have met, you will already have a preconceived idea of who they are. Thus, is the power and beauty of perfume and your sense of smell.

the ancient Egyptians

Perfume-makers in ancient Egypt were very highly regarded and usually members of religious orders. It was the duty of a priest to mix the aromatic spices and herbs for the incense that would be burned in a temple. The potency of ground and mulled aromatics like myrrh, sandalwood, cypresswood, and frankincense to create an atmosphere of magical and religious intent was not underestimated. Incense or perfumes used in the worship of royalty or gods were regarded as ecclesiastical mysteries and their recipes were

above: **Note the perfume cones on this fresco of ancient Egyptian dancers.**

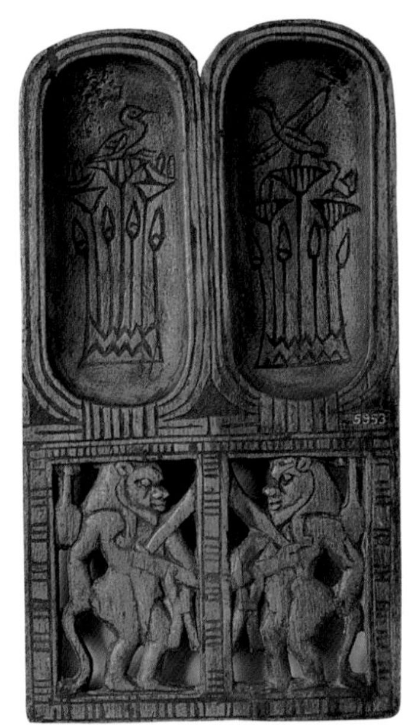

above: **Ointment Spoon decorated with plants and birds, c.1300 BC.**

right: **Hippocrates, Greek philosopher and medic.**

secret, passed like priceless heirlooms from father to son.

Perfumes were not solely confined to religious rituals; they were used for bathing by all members of society. The ancient Egyptians reveled in the pleasures of the bath and were renowned for their fastidious approach to hygiene and their penchant for using cosmetics to freshen and enhance their bodies. Even though the oils and ointments that were used by the masses were far inferior to those that were rubbed and pummeled into the bodies of the nobility, the masses took their perfumes seriously. Apparently, during the reign of Pharaoh Seti I, soldiers were rewarded by increases in their allocation of aromatic oils, and gravediggers once went on strike because their ration of food and oils was to be cut.

Perfumed oils and aromatic substances also found their way into medicine cabinets. There was a general belief that certain strong-smelling substances of vegetable origin had antiseptic qualities, and that flowers and aromatic gums, oils, and resins could be utilized to prevent disease. In the Papyrus Ebers, dated about 1800 BC, in a document called *The Sacred Perfume of Kyptri*, a formula for fumigating and perfuming a house or clothing for sanitary purposes was given. It lists the ingredients as myrrh, juniper, frankincense, cypresswood, aloeswood, mastic, and styrax.

The ingredients used in the manufacture of perfumes in ancient Egypt were, of course, derived from completely natural materials. While many locally available flowers and plants were used, some came from distant lands. Because of this, certain perfumes were a precious commodity that could only be made in minute quantities, their value exceeding that of silver and gold. Understandably no expense was spared when it came to storing perfume, and only the most beautiful containers were thought appropriate.

It is from the ancient Egyptians that the original notion of perfumes as luxury items is possibly derived. So esteemed were they that spices, for example, were among the gifts that the Queen of Sheba presented to King Solomon.

the ancient Greeks

According to legend the Elysian Fields—the Greek idea of heaven—were filled with perfume. The gates to its golden city were made of cinnamon, its fountains sprayed water of sweet essences, and

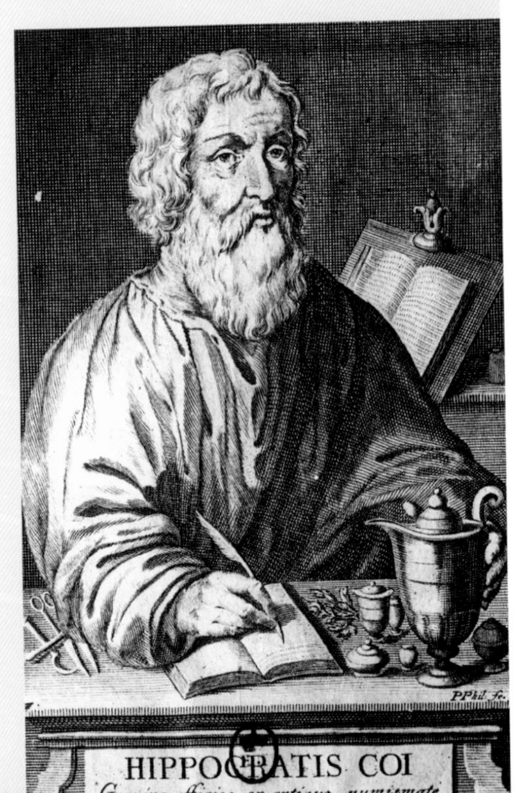

through the city ran a river of perfume that enveloped everything in a mist of fragrant dew. Though the Egyptians took their perfumes seriously, one cannot doubt the enthusiasm of the Greeks who endowed the plants used for perfume-making with divine origins and even named some of them in honor of their gods and goddesses.

Perfume was so well regarded that perfume shops began to function as meeting places for philosophers and statesmen who would argue and discuss the subtleties of individual perfumes. The great Greek philosopher and medic Hippocrates, recommended the use of perfumes to promote good health. He wrote that "the best-known recipe for health is to apply sweet scents unto the brain." Pliny and Dioscorides, both classical authors, wrote about the cultivation of aromatic plants and the production of ointments and perfumes.

The use of perfume was widespread and not simply the domain of the chattering classes, but there were some who frowned on its use. A few conservative and powerful citizens saw it as a self-indulgence that was not to be encouraged, so in a few of the Italian states perfume became a prohibited item.

the ancient Hebrews

In this culture, aromatic spices and resins were used for symbolic rituals in the temples and in medicine, rather than for personal adornment or indulgence. The priests so feared that perfume would be used for profane purposes that perfume recipes and the methods of its manufacture were closely guarded secrets. Hebrew women were forbidden to wear or carry perfume except on the Sabbath, when they were permitted to carry camures—gold or silver hollow globes filled with perfume—and then only with the intention of warding off ill health.

Because of this strictly regulated use of aromatics, a black market in perfumes flourished. Most of these artful sales were made in an area of old Jerusalem—called the Old Spice Market—that was also the meeting place for women of the night who used perfumes in abundance. This conjunction of perfume, prostitutes, and illegal trading served only to fortify the belief among religious elders that perfume was indeed ruinous to moral decency.

the ancient Romans

The most decadent users of perfume were the Romans who, like the Greeks, thought it fashionable to rendezvous in *unguentani*, the perfume shops, for a spot of socializing among the scented cream of Roman society. But if the great and good were not to be found in the perfume shops, then they would surely be pleasuring themselves in the communal baths. In these elaborate public bathing places, one room—the unctuarium—was devoted entirely to storing perfumed oils and ointments.

Many stories have been told of how the Romans were lavish in their use of perfumes. Men

above: **Clay oil burner from Roman times.**

would often wear different perfumes on different parts of their bodies and perfume each of their garments separately. Even their horses and dogs would be rubbed down with aromatic oils. In the houses of the wealthy, beds and couches were stuffed to overflowing with dried flowers, and guests at banquets would be given gold or alabaster containers of perfume.

One of the best stories of opulence and extravagance concerns how the wings of caged doves were saturated with perfume and the birds where then released so that fragrance would rain down upon the heads of guests and revelers.

The perfume industry flourished and standards of perfume refinement reached unprecedented levels. Naturally, the profession of perfume-maker was a highly regarded one and it was said that "Happy is he whose craft is that of a perfume-maker." Although sources list the uses of perfumes and some basic methods of preparation, virtually no recipes were recorded. This is probably because they were family secrets, passed verbally from generation to generation.

HOW THE OILS WERE EXTRACTED

pressing

This is one of the oldest known methods; the Egyptians depicted the pressing process in wall paintings that were uncovered in archeological digs. Fragrant plants were crushed in a basin, in much the same way as grapes were pressed to make wine. The crushed material was placed on a cloth, which was then folded. Rods were threaded through loops at either end of the cloth and then turned in opposite directions to twist the cloth into a tight bundle. As the cloth tightened, oils were released from the crushed plants.

cold steeping

This process, which later became known as enfleurage, was particularly suitable for extracting the oil from petals. The petals were laid onto a layer of animal fat and then pressed between two boards. When the petal scent had been absorbed by the fat, these petals were thrown away and fresh petals sprinkled over the fat. This process continued for several weeks until the fat was totally permeated with scent. The resulting pomade was strained and then washed in a preserving wine or alcohol solution.

maceration

A jar containing a mixture of oil or fat, astringent wine, and water was preheated in large vats of boiling water—an arrangement that is very much like our modern-day double-boiler. Resins or plant materials were steeped in the liquid that was heated to about 150 degrees Fahrenheit. The mixture was left to stand for several days before being agitated and strained. This method has remained largely unchanged for thousand of years and is still regarded as basic perfume-making.

THE INGREDIENTS

♥

"A caravan from China comes,
For miles it sweetens all the air
With fragrant silks and stealing gums
Attar and Myrrh—
A caravan from China comes.
O merchant, tell me what you bring,
With music sweet of camel bells,
How long have you been travelling
With these sweet smells?
O merchant, tell me what you bring."

♥

Many of the plants and spices that were used in perfume-making in ancient times were indigenous to China, Hindustan, and Persia. As trade increased and the Silk Route was opened, so did the availability of exotic and rare scents. Caravans of traders would travel for months to bring their wares into Arabia and Egypt and into the hands of the Greeks and Romans.

Perfume ingredients mentioned in ancient manuscripts are: aloeswood, ambergris, angelica, basil, benzoin gum, camphor, canella bark, citron peel, cloves, coriander, cedar bark, cinnamon, cypress, jasmine, juniper, lavender, mace, marjoram, mint, musk, myrrh, myrtle, nutmeg, olibanum (frankincense), orange blossom, orris root, peony root, quince peel, rosemary, rose leaves, saffron, sandalwood, spikenard, styrax, thyme, valerian, violets, and water lilies. Reading through this scented roll-call makes one realize that many of the ingredients of modern perfumes have been used since the history of perfume was first recorded. While some, for example musk and ambergris, can no longer be used in their natural form, they have been chemically reinvented.

Here are stories behind some of the more exotic scents that hailed from the Far East and were carried along the Silk Route.

Ambergris—or attar as it is known in Arabic, was originally the name given to any perfume, but was later used only to describe the perfume derived from "the biliary concretion in the intestines of the sperm whale." The sperm whale once ranged throughout "all the seven seas," and was hunted down by whalers from Brazil to Madagascar, the East Indies to Africa. The slaughter of sperm whales is now virtually a criminal offence so the ambergris fragrance is synthetically created in perfume laboratories.

Jasmine—for many years associated with romance and indigenous to the ancient fertile lands of Persia, it is now cultivated in almost every corner of the world. Kama, the Hindu god of love, tipped his arrows with jasmine blossoms so that they would pierce hearts with desire.

Musk—made from a secretion of the male musk deer of the Himalayas, it was for hundreds of years used solely by the Indians and Chinese, until it, too, found its way into the perfume shops of Arabia and the West. Musk is very symbolic for Muslims who believe that Paradise is fragrant with its heavy, sweet, and exotic smell. In fact, the

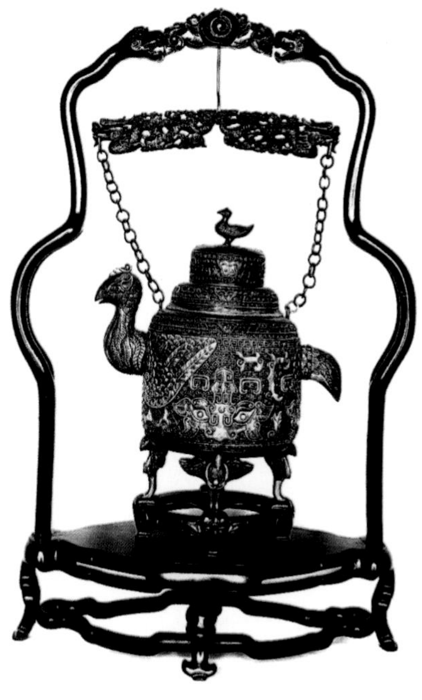

above: **Old Chinese oil burner.**

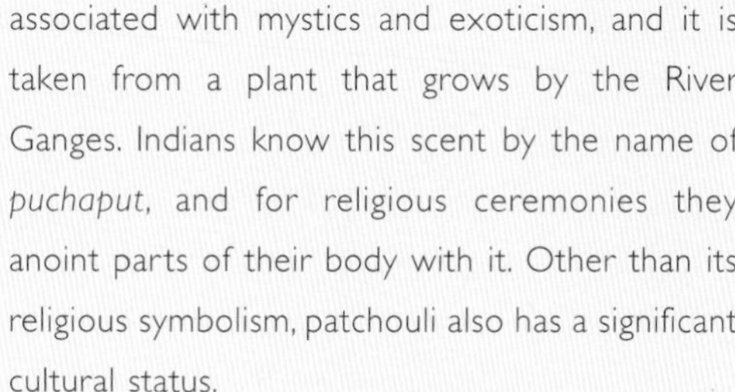

mortar used in the construction of ancient mosques was mixed with musk so that its aroma constantly filled the air.

Modern perfumes use a synthetic musk that mimics the rare and natural original. In these days of environmental concern and wildlife preservation, the hunting of the musk deer purely for its scent is frowned upon.

Patchouli—this heavy and musky fragrance is often associated with mystics and exoticism, and it is taken from a plant that grows by the River Ganges. Indians know this scent by the name of *puchaput*, and for religious ceremonies they anoint parts of their body with it. Other than its religious symbolism, patchouli also has a significant cultural status.

Rose water—first distilled by the Arabian doctor and chemist Avicenna in the eleventh century, from the rose *Rosa centfolia*. When Sultan Saladin conquered Jerusalem in 1187 he ordered that rose water be mixed into the mortar being used for the floors and walls of mosques. It was introduced to Europe by Crusaders returning from Jerusalem and Arabia and was initially used in finger bowls. It was not long before rose water became a staple ingredient in cosmetics and cleansers, and as a perfume in its own right. Rose water is still used as a skin tonic.

Saffron—even in modern times saffron, produced from the stamens of the crocus flower, is still regarded as an incredibly valuable substance. Cultivated in Persia and used for many centuries in China and India, it was praised for its heavenly scent and for its culinary and medical applications. Legend has it that the only tears ever shed by a crocodile fell when the crocodile inhaled the fragrance of saffron in a field of crocuses.

Sandalwood—there are records of its use in perfume-making dating from 500 BC, but historians agree that it was probably in use much earlier. Sandalwood is produced from the sap of an Indian tree and it is considered to be sacred in many cultures. It was an object of worship for

below: **Etching of Catherine de' Medici, who popularized the perfumed glove.**

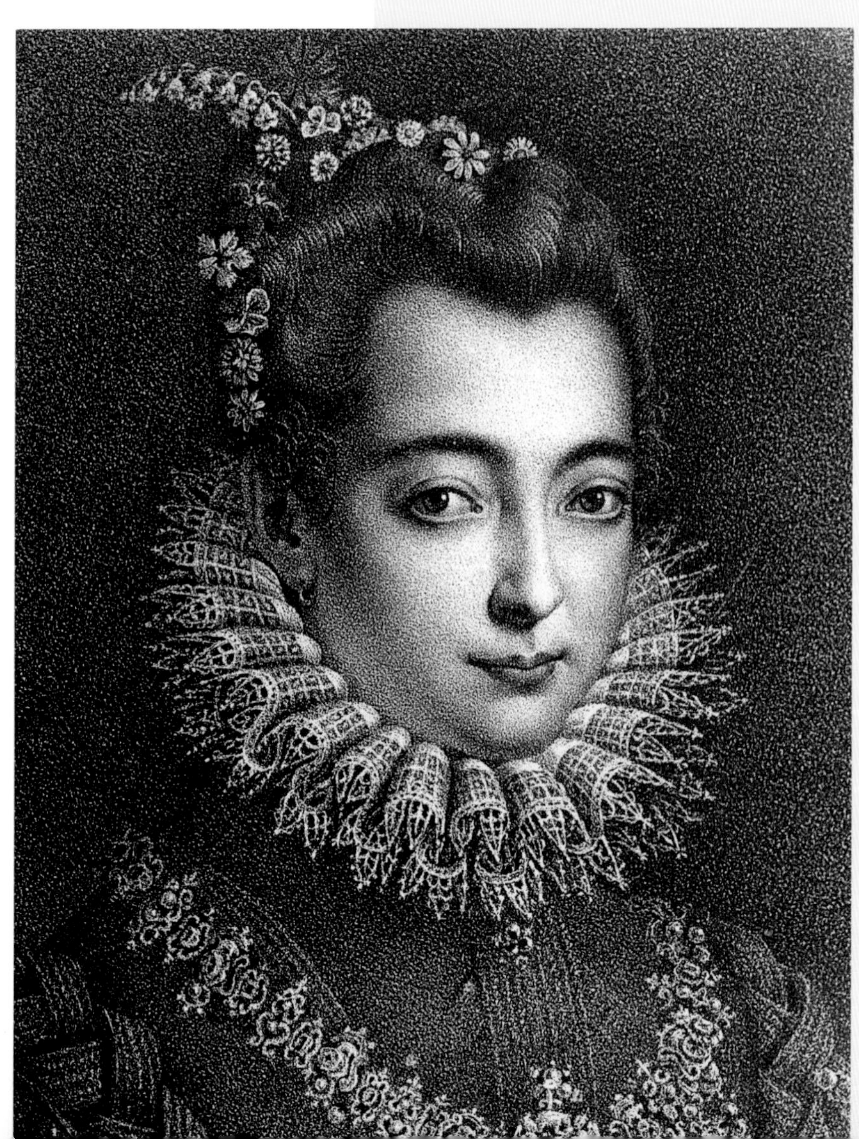

Indian Hindus, Chinese Buddhists, and many ancient cultures of Africa.

Spikenard—used in numerous ancient perfume compounds, the spikenard plant is a member of the valerian family that grows in Bhutan and Nepal. There is a wonderful story about how the army of Alexander the Great was overcome by its fragrance when spikenard plants were crushed beneath the feet of Alexander's elephants.

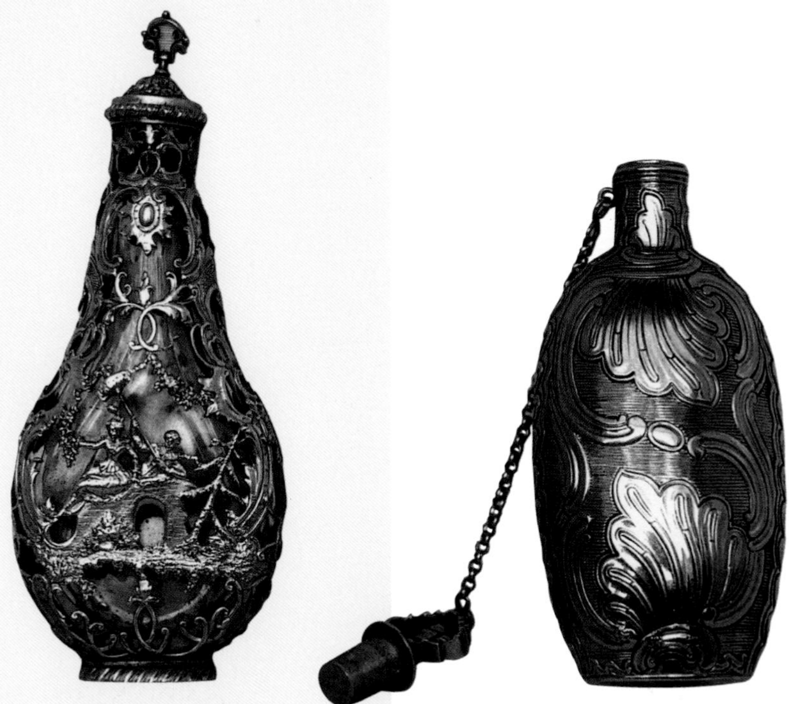

above: **French Regency perfume bottle.**

above left: **French Louis XV perfume bottle with ornate gold chasing.**

perfume making in the west

Once the art of perfume making reached France in the twelfth century, the industry became a force to be reckoned with, achieving a popularity not experienced since the heady days of ancient Rome. In 1190, in one of his earliest acts, King Philip II (also known as Philip Augustus) granted a charter for the perfumers of Paris. This amounted to a royal seal that resulted in perfume being added to anything—clothes, cosmetics, furnishings, and bedding.

All the rage during the early fifteenth century were tiny satin sachets, called *coussines*, that were filled with lavender and violet. King Charles VI had many of them made for his beloved Queen Isabeau of Bavaria, who being more than a modest perfume indulger herself had her rooms at the palace scented with *oislette de chypre*. *Oislette de chypre* were little decorative birds made of silk and covered with feathers, and filled with perfumed powders.

Catherine de' Medici, wife of Henry II of France, had her own personal perfumer, Rene le Florentine, whom she shared with her son, Henry III. According to historical manuscripts and paintings, the young Henry liked to make up his face with powders and cosmetics—the finished look being very feminine—and had a preference for perfume concoctions that dated back to the boudoir of Nero's wife, Poppoea.

Catherine's perfumer was responsible for the invention of the perfumed glove that was extremely fashionable for many years on both sides of the English Channel. Le Florentine's creation turned the perfume industry upside-down, and until the reign of Louis XIV perfume industry sales were a branch of the glove manufacturers'. In 1656 this was changed by a charter that created the Guild of Gautiers-perfumeurs.

When Queen Elizabeth I was presented with a pair of perfumed gloves, she delighted in them. For not only were they beautiful, they made it

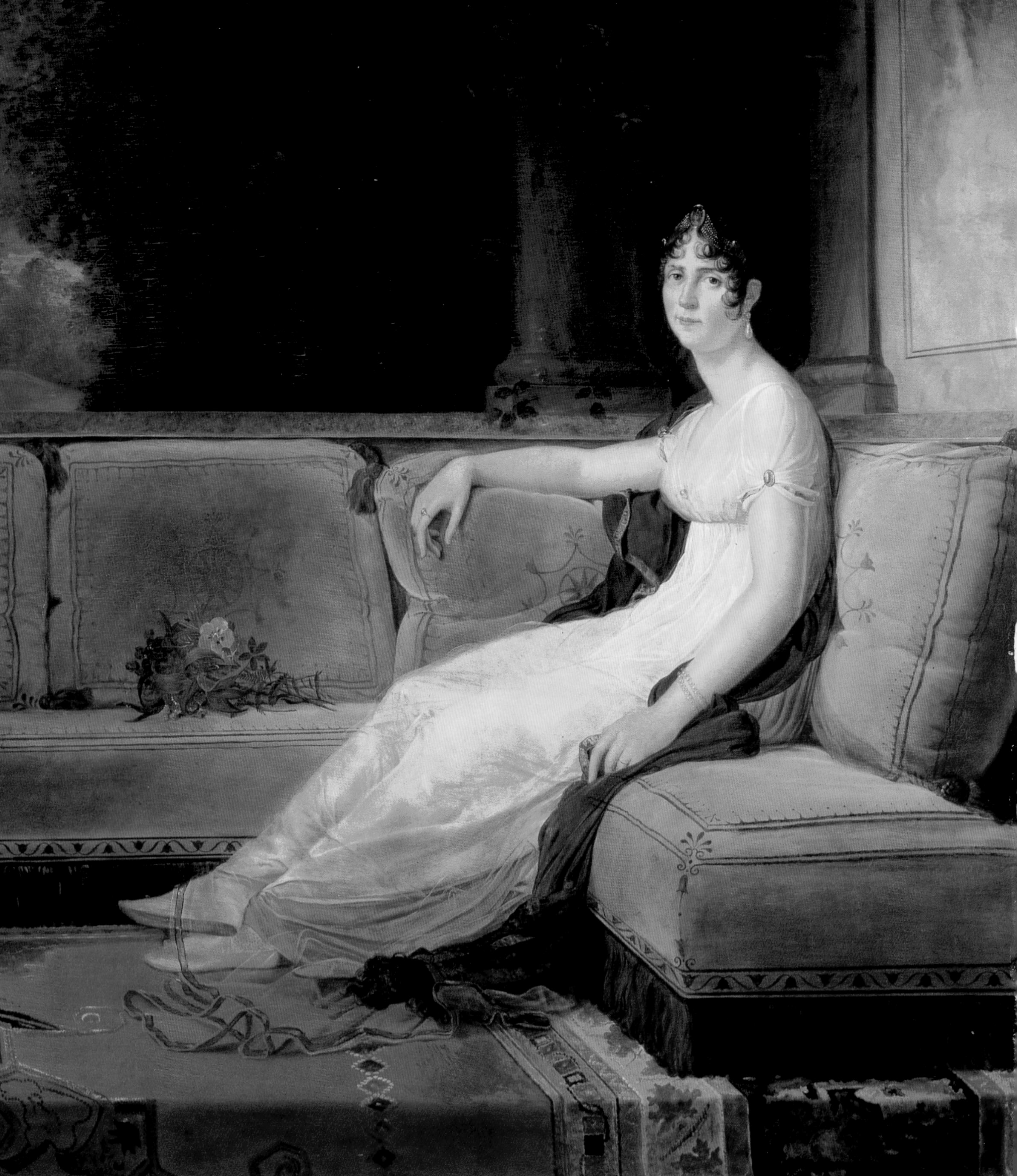

easy for her to block terrible odors by simply placing a gloved hand to her nose. During Elizabeth's reign pomanders were also popular. They were used to disguise stenches and thought to be a preventive measure against disease.

Pomanders were compounds of dried aromatic substances that were mixed into a paste and placed into small spherical containers suitable for carrying. Pomanders were originally called *pomme d'embre*. *Pomme*, the French for apple, aptly describing the spherical container, and with *d'embre* indicating that ambergris was an ingredient in the scented compound. Elizabeth took great pleasure in the art of perfume and was known to compose her own fragrances using apples, aromatic substances, and curiously "the fat of a young dog!"

The perfume bubble burst for a short time during the reign of Louis XIV. Once known as "the Sweet Smelling Monarch," Louis decided that his intense migraines were caused by his perfumes and he banished perfume from his courts. The only perfume exempted from his decree was orange blossom. Louis' ban was taken seriously by his courtiers, so much so that "the court ladies pretended to faint away at the sight of a flower," records the diary of a Sicilian visitor.

By the time of his death and the subsequent reign of Louis XV, a decadent and frivolous monarch, perfumes were enjoying a fashionable resurgence. Louis XV used a different perfume every day, and his mistress—the infamous Madame Pompadour—was also extravagant in her use of scents. In one year her perfume bill amounted to five hundred thousand livres, or about one hundred thousand dollars!

Madame Pompadour's extravagance was taken to ridiculous extremes by the flamboyant and narcissistic ladies and gentlemen of the French nobility who piled perfume upon perfume on their bodies and garments, and layer-upon-layer of powder on their faces and wigs.

Even Napoleon's wife, the Empress Josephine, had an enormous penchant for perfumes, which she had sent from Martinique. It is said that her chambers were so saturated with musk that even sixty years after her death, it still penetrated the air with its heavy fragrance.

By the turn of the nineteenth century, not only was "la toilette" a time-consuming daily ritual, it was an institution with many books devoted to the subject of cosmetics. Experts expounded widely and loudly on definitions of beauty, and shared their formulas for potions and perfumes.

Technical and chemical innovations during the late nineteenth century revolutionized the perfume industry and set it on the path that it travels today (see pages 24 to 27). According to recent figures, the perfume industry in the U.S. is worth about sixty million dollars a year. Perfumes are available to everyone and they are worn by people from all walks of life. We no longer ration our perfumes by saving them for special occasions, we apply them daily as part of our toilette and dressing routine.

While the perfumers have taken every advantage of synthesized essences, some of the best-selling perfumes use recipes that are up to

left: ***Josephine at Malmaison*, by François Gerard.**

two hundred years old. *Creed* was first produced in 1760, *Guerlain* (Guerlain) in 1828, and *Molinard* in 1849. This simply goes to show that even though technology has caught up with perfumes, the appeal and mysticism of perfume is as old as human civilization.

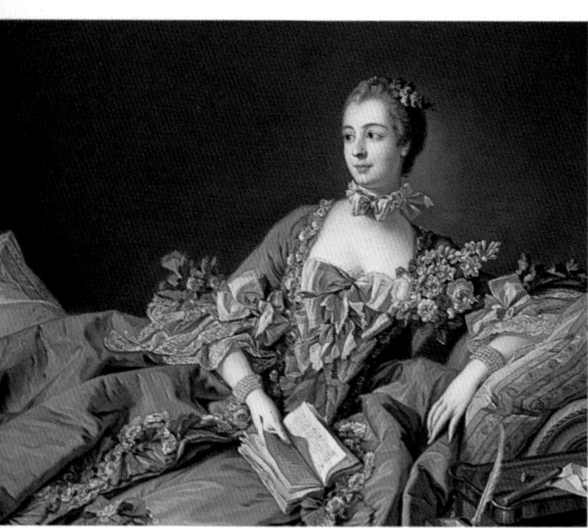

above: ***Madame de Pompadour*** **by the French artist François Boucher.**

right: **The launch of *Miss Balmain* in Paris, 1967.**

perfume between the covers

One of the earliest books on perfumes was *Les Secrets de Maistre Alexys le Liedmontois* which was published in the sixteenth century. While much of the text is as one would expect, there are some unusual moments. One of these is the rather frightening recipe for "magical water"— "Take a young raven from the nest, feed it on hard eggs for forty days, kill it and distil it with myrtle leaves, talc and almond oil."

Le Perfumeur François, which was published in 1693 and written by Simon Barbe, is a teaching manual that describes the various methods of extracting the scent from flowers and of preparing all kinds of perfumes. One of the secrets it shares with its readers is how to perfume tobacco. Barbe intended that his book would be "For the entertainment of the nobility, the use of religious purposes and indispensable to bath house keepers and hairdressers."

Published in 1925, *The Closet of Beauty, or an old way to procure new loveliness* used extracts from a seventeenth-century book *The Ladies Dictionary*. Among its "fragrant recipes and much quaint advice" on making perfumed formulas and scented bracelets, it has this to say about boxes of perfume— "Boxes are very necessary on Sunday occasions, viz. To hinder Vapors, prevent infections, remove ill scents, or bad Airs ..." Apparently these boxes were filled with an aromatic compound that could protect ladies "against the plague, pestilence and cold" yet be "pleasant and delightful to the Brain."

Another beauty encyclopedia, this one written by Arnold J. Cobley in the nineteenth century, gives a description of eau de Cologne—"A favorite and fashionable scent for personal use and the one most extensively employed. It is also used as a cosmetic, to remove freckles, acne, etc. A very large quantity is likewise consumed by ladies, in the high life, as a cordial and stimulant to drive away vapors and perfume the breath... A piece of linen dipped in Eau de Cologne and laid across the forehead or on the temples, is the fashionable remedy for a nervous headache..."

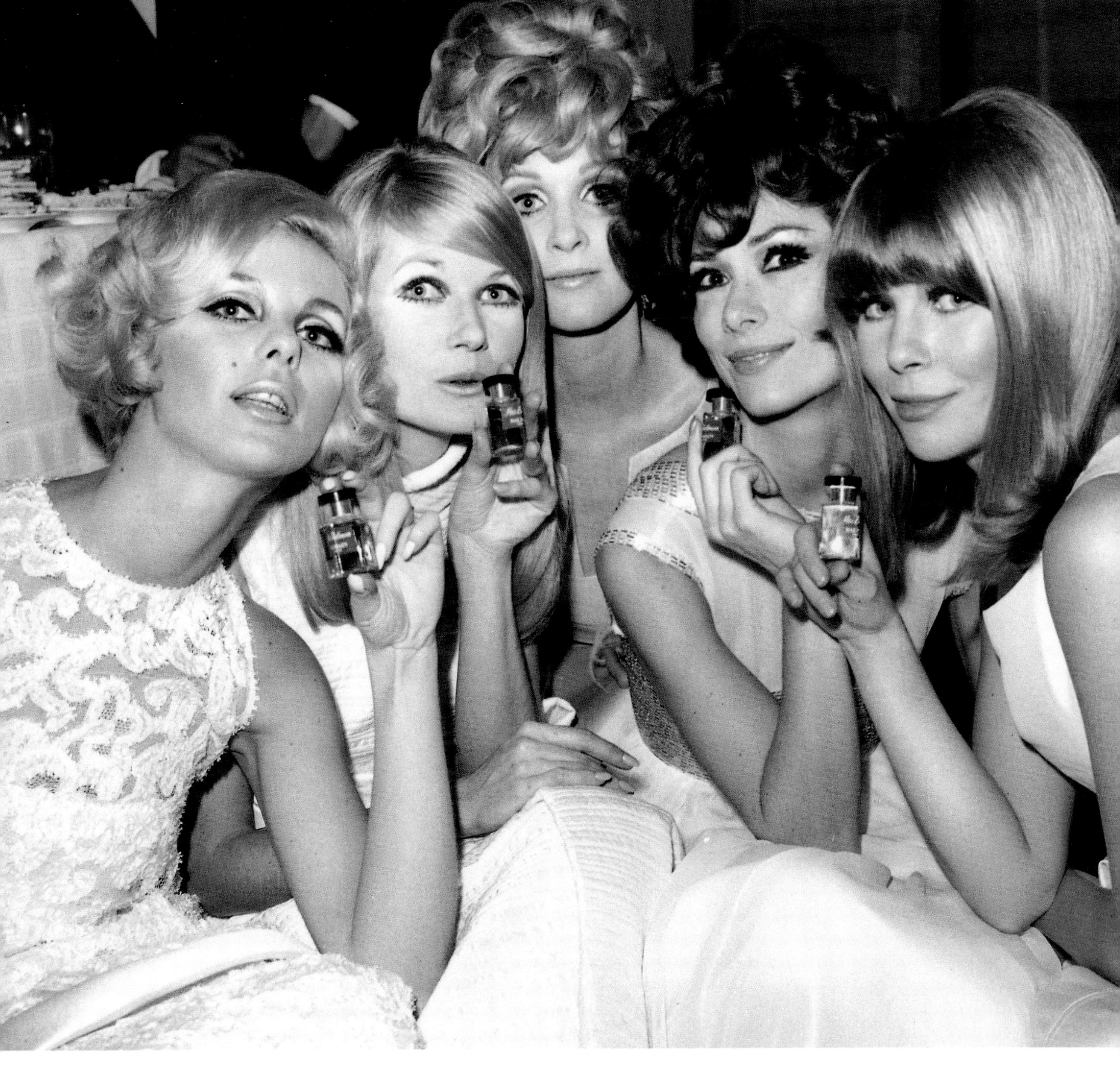

2

chapter

the perf

di

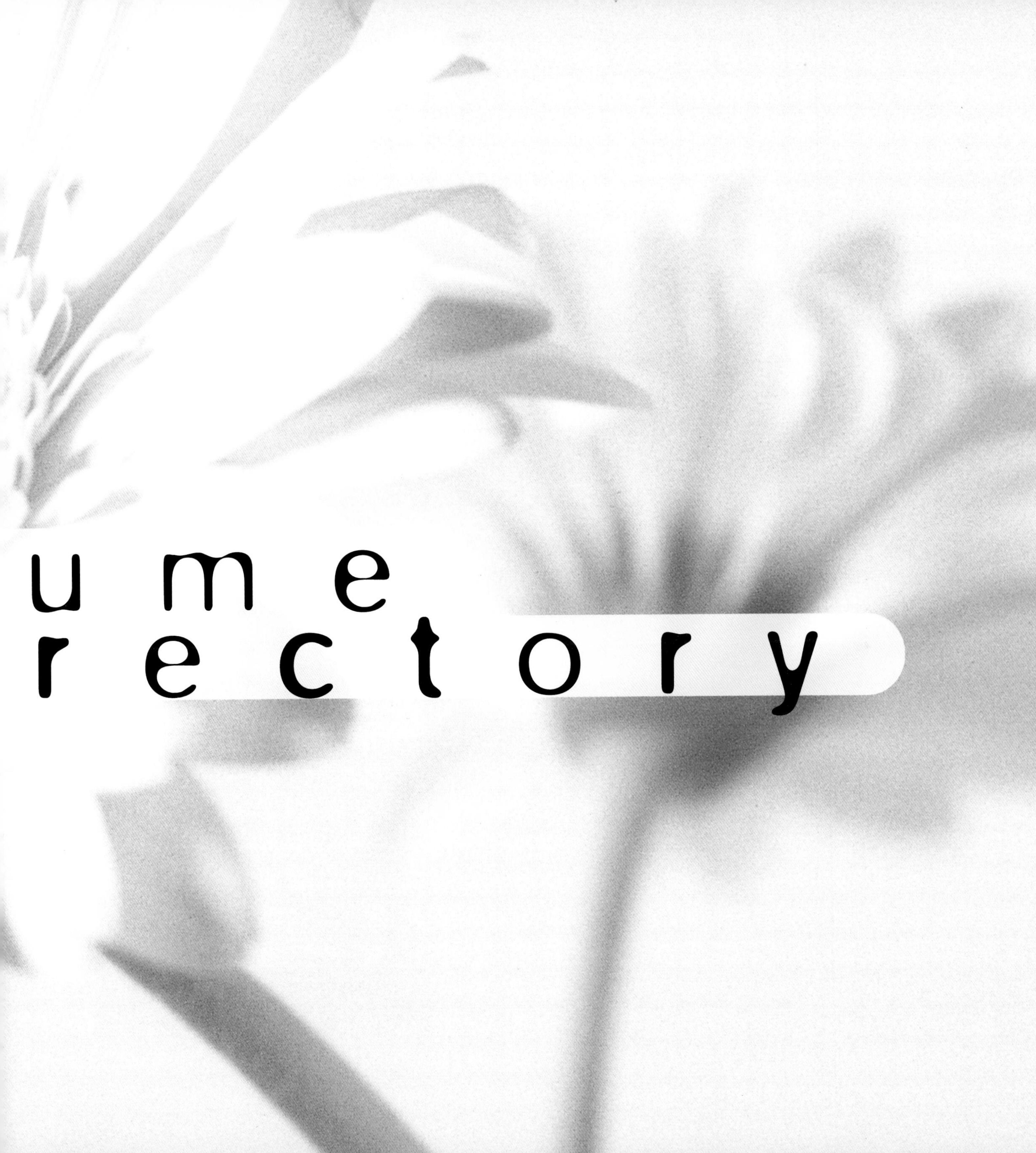
ume
rectory

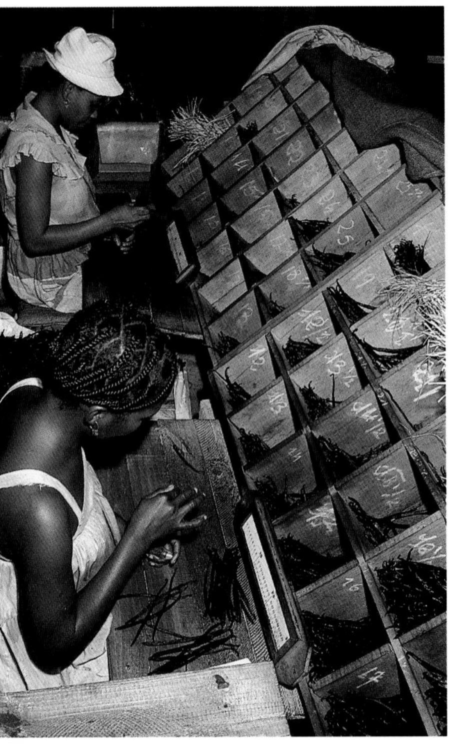

above: **Grading vanilla in Northeast Madagascar.**

right: **Orange blossom—the plant from which neroli oil is derived.**

In our search for the ultimate scent many perfumes have been developed over the last century. The natural world has been an orchard of blossoms and fragrances from which the most divine of species have been tenderly harvested by perfumers, their scents patiently caressed to create perfumes of extraordinary variety.

Developments in technology have lead to progress in the methods used to distill perfume. The initial and most important stage in the manufacture of perfume is the extraction of the essential oils from plants by enfleurage, expression, steam distillation, or by chemical solvents.

enfleurage

Enfleurage, which was used from the time of the ancient Egyptians until the beginning of the twentieth century, extracts the essential oils or "absoluts" by saturating an animal fat with the scent of plants and flowers. Animal fat, preserved with gum benzoin tincture, was smeared onto a framed plate and plants or flowers were sprinkled onto it and left to release their oils. The plants or flowers were removed and replaced daily until the fat was completely saturated with the scent.

This pomade was then mixed with alcohol (the ancient Egyptians used wine), heated and then cooled until all the essential oils were dissolved into the alcohol. The concoction was filtered to remove the plant mass and the fat. The alcohol was then evaporated to leave the absolut—the purest form of perfume that retains most of the plant's aromatic constituents.

Because enfleurage was a time-consuming ritual, the resulting absolut was extremely expensive and very rare. An absolut of jasmine, for example, could cost in the region of $27,000 for about two pounds. This method is hardly used nowadays, but small amounts of enfleurage-extracted absoluts are used by manufacturers like Chanel and Guerlain.

expression

This method is used to extract essential oils from fruits, especially citrus fruits. The technique involves cold pressing the rinds between rollers and sponges to remove the oils.

steam distillation

The is the most popular way of extracting essential oils and it has been in use in Arabic countries for about 5000 years, though many centuries passed before it was introduced to the West.

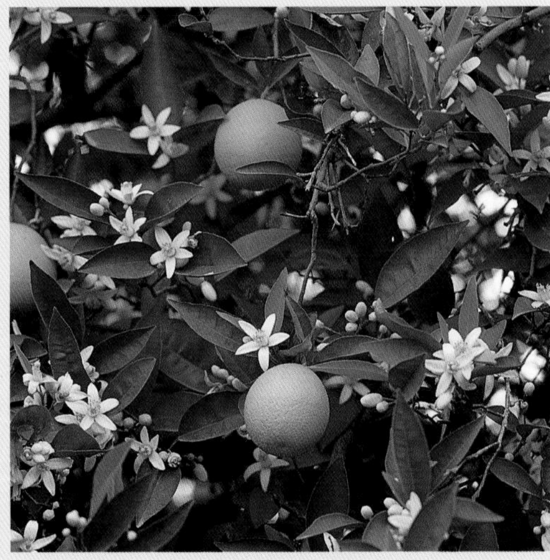

In steam distillation, plants are boiled in water in a vessel called an alembic. The steam, saturated with the essential oil, rises from the boiling mixture and is collected in a pipe which is connected to another vessel. The steam then condenses into liquid form with the oil floating on the top of the water.

One of the few improvements to this technique involves laying plants on grill-like racks and passing intensely heated steam through them. The advantage of this development is that every last molecule of the essential oil is extracted.

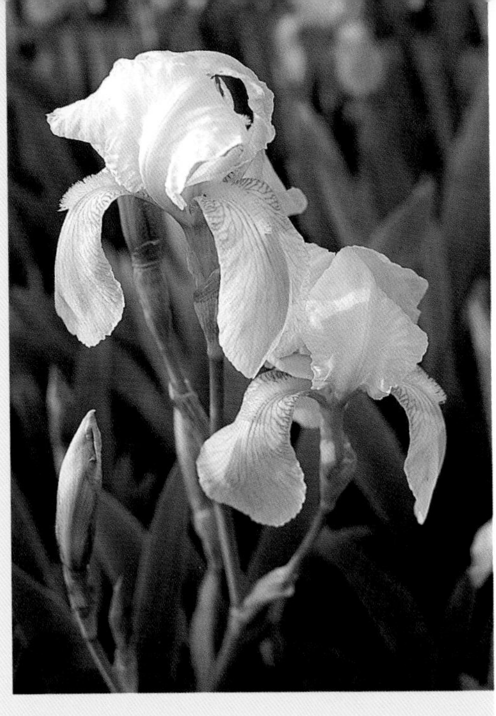

left: **The orris plant in bloom.**

chemical solvents

To extract very delicate fragrances from some flowers, chemical solvents are used. If steam distillation was used in such instances, the extreme heat would damage the fragrance.

The process involves placing the flowers onto the perforated metal layers of a huge extractor into which solvents are piped. The solvents and flowers are then heated gently until the flowers' essential oils, vegetable waxes, and pigments are dissolved into the solvent. This combination is boiled in an alembic to evaporate the solvent. The concrete left behind is a solid mixture of essence and wax. The wax is removed by mixing the concrete with alcohol and then passing it through a filter to separate out the wax. The resulting liquid is heated again to evaporate the alcohol, leaving behind the pure essential oil.

There are many stories about the flowers and plants that are used in perfume manufacture.

Neroli—is derived from the flowers of orange trees grown in the south of France, southern Spain, Italy, and North Africa. The orange blossom, as it is otherwise known, has a sweet and intense aroma and has been a symbol of fertility for years. Arab brides wore the flower and this tradition passed into Christian practice with the Crusades. Many of today's brides continue this tradition by including orange blossoms in their bouquet. The orange blossom was named after an Italian princess who made it fashionable in the seventeenth century to scent gloves with their fragrance.

Orris—is derived from the dried root of the iris plant. Its scent is soft, deep, and powdery and harmonizes with the natural scent of the human body. Because of this affinity, orris is regarded as an aphrodisiac. Orris has been a much-loved perfume since Greek times, was named in honor of the Greek goddess of the rainbow, and was regarded as a symbol of kingship. To extract the perfume from the flower, orris bulbs are stored and dried on wooden shelves for up to two years, then powdered and continually steam distilled over a period of six months. The yield from this labor is just a tiny amount of essential oil.

Rose oil—and rose water have been used for thousands of years and fossils of wild roses have been discovered that date back as far as forty million years. The Persians were probably the first to distill rose water and were responsible for exporting it across the world until the Middle Ages.

There are many different kinds of roses, but rose essential oils come from two main species—the cabbage rose that has a light and crisp fragrance, and the heavier-scented damask rose. The damask rose was used widely by the Arabs, who were among the first to discover its ambrosial scent. More than half the perfumes that we wear today use rose oil.

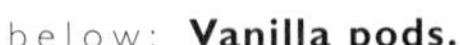

below: **Vanilla pods.**

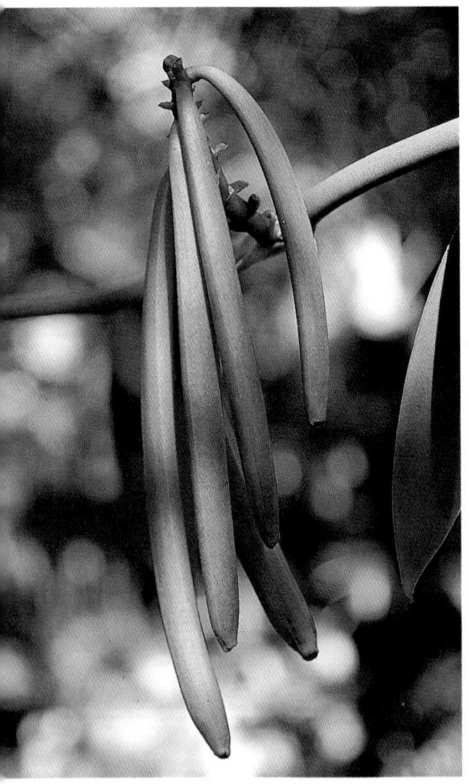

Vanilla—was discovered as a perfume in about 1520 in Mexico. Until that time the Aztecs had enjoyed it as a flavoring in chocolate drinks. The vanilla pods are put through a six-month fermenting and drying process that ends only when the essential oil-bearing white crystals appear on the pods. Many modern-day perfumes contain the soft, fondant scent of vanilla, although it is often a synthetic vanilla that is used.

Ylang-ylang—means "the flower of flowers" and its perfume has been valued for hundreds if not thousands of years throughout Southeast Asia where it is grown in the Philippines, Madagascar, and Java. Ylang-ylang has an exotic and richly sweet fragrance that is only apparent in the mature flower. To capture their ephemeral scent, the flowers have to be gathered very quickly.

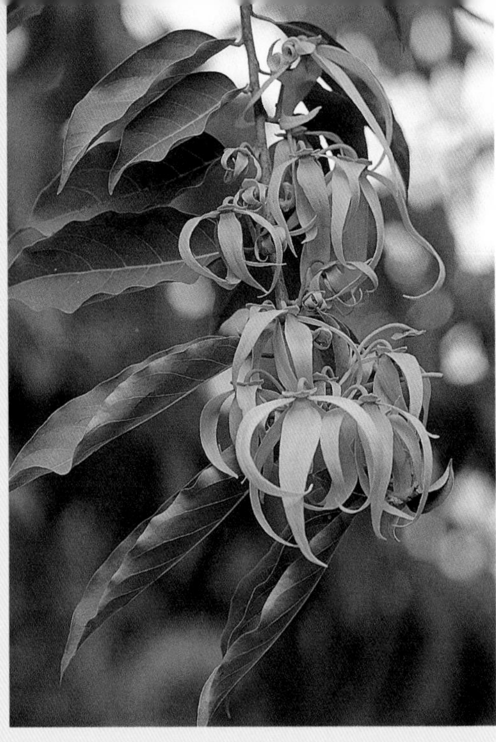

above: **Ylang-ylang flower.**

synthetic essences

Because of the cost and rarity of true essence, many perfumes are made using a synthetic equivalent. But before you lambaste perfume manufacturers, you must appreciate that without synthetic ingredients most of the world's most popular perfumes could not have been created. Though the synthetic versions of the true essences cannot hold a candle to the delight of the natural essences—some lacking the subtlety and variety of notes of the originals—they are under constant development, the aim of which is to replicate the smell of the originals so that they affect our olfactory nerves in exactly the same way.

The method of synthesizing aromatic compositions was developed in 1877 by Friedel, a Frenchman, and Crafts, an American. It is accepted that this date marks the birth of the modern perfume industry.

The work of these two men totally revolutionized the way perfumes were made. Before 1877, massive quantities of raw materials were required to make minimal amounts of essential oils. It took, for example, 250 pounds of oranges to produce just one ounce of orange essence. Gone also was the labor-intensive and time-consuming, and therefore expensive, process of extracting the essential oils. Synthetics also meant that the manufacturers and users of perfumes were not prey to the vagaries of nature that could destroy thousands of acres of plants and flowers and send prices soaring. Chemical counterparts also meant that quality control could be monitored and kept constant, and that new combinations of fragrances could be easily and relatively inexpensively tried and tested. Such luxuries were not afforded to earlier perfumers.

The greatest result of this revolution was that the world of perfumes became accessible to a whole new class of people—the perfume industry hit boom time. If one thinks of scent in terms of being a concoction of chemicals, then the very essences of true perfumes are themselves natural chemicals. Therefore many of the ingredients found in the synthetic creations are identical to those found in nature. There are two forms of synthetic perfumes.

The first are the isolates. These are the chemicals that are individually separated out from essential oils and used in the manufacture of perfume. Perhaps it is fair to say that these chemicals are more natural than synthetic.

The second type of synthetics is actually produced by chemical reactions that involve petroleum and coal tar. Because the fragrances of some plants and flowers cannot be extracted in sufficient quantities, the creation of a totally synthetic version is the only way that these fragrances ever make it to the perfume counter. In the trial-and-error process of trying to recreate nature's bountiful aromas, many original and extraordinary scents have been created in laboratories around the world.

The search to capture and synthesize the more elusive natural fragrances has meant that new techniques have been developed. One of these involves passing carbon dioxide in a suspended state (somewhere between being a liquid and a gas) through the plant or flower. This freeze-dries the raw material, locking in the fragrance. Unlike enfleurage or distillation, soft extraction does not alter the natural scent in any way. It should come as no surprise, then, that this is the method used to extract the coffee flavor from coffee beans and so make instant freeze-dried coffee.

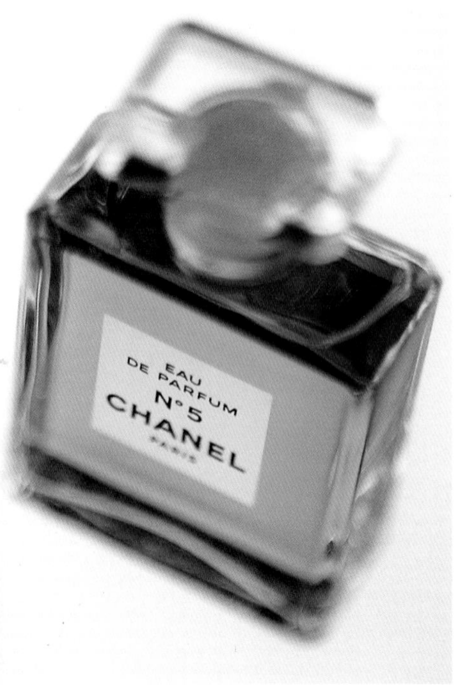

eau de chocolate, anyone?

The scents of coffee and chocolate have recently been incorporated in some perfumes. As we all know, chocolate is renowned for its aphrodisiac qualities and it has been chemically proven that it induces the giddy and euphoric feelings we succumb to when falling in love. Casanova knew this because his favorite nightcap was hot chocolate spiced up with another sexy scent, ambergris resin. The use, therefore, of chocolate in the perfume industry as the absolute ultimate fragrance of seduction seems quite natural. Two contemporary perfumes that use chocolate bass notes are Thierry Mugler's *Angel* and Coty's *Ici*.

The perfume house of Caron was once commissioned by an American billionaire to make a perfume that was to smell like champagne. The billionaire, apparently, was in the habit of bathing in the stuff. The result was "Royal Bain de Champagne." Almost any fragrance can be recreated for the purpose of perfume. Donna Karan had one of her favorite smells, which happened to be from a famous Fifth Avenue tobacconist, recreated for her scent *DK Man*.

two perfumes of note

We cannot talk about perfumes without mentioning the two most famous scents of the twentieth century, Chanel *No. 5* and Jean Patou's *Joy*.

No. 5 was created in 1921 by Chanel's "nose," Ernest Beaux. It was developed during a time when couturiers found that creating a scent for their fashion houses heightened their fame and added a certain panache to their name. Never one to miss an opportunity, Coco Chanel asked Beaux to create a fragrance for her. Beaux duly delivered two batches of perfumes, numbered from 1 to 5 and 20 to 24 for Coco to try. Perfume number five was not her first choice, but five was, for Coco, a significant number. From when she was a child in an orphanage she had remembered the patterned figure of number five that had decorated the floor near her room.

Chanel *No. 5* is a concoction of jasmine, orris root, neroli, and vanilla, plus a synthetic compound called aldehyde, which mimics a chemical that occurs naturally in the human skin. This resulted in a unique perfume—aldehyde smells nothing like anything in nature, but has a warmth and resonance that is immediately appealing.

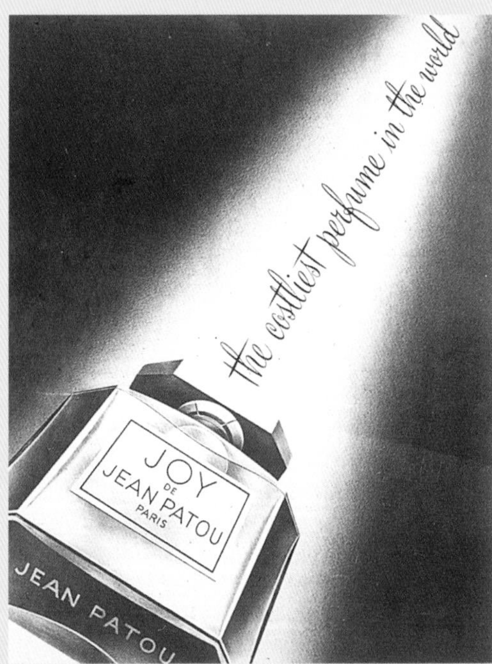

above: **No. 5 by Chanel has been one of the most enduring scents of the twentieth century.**

right: **Sales of *Joy* by Jean Patou confirmed that no price is too high for perfume.**

The most famous user of *No. 5* was the ultimate sex symbol, Marilyn Monroe. When asked what she wore in bed, Marilyn famously replied, "The only thing I wear in bed is Chanel *No. 5*." Sales of *No. 5* rocketed and it has remained at the top ever since.

Joy was made for the house of Jean Patou in 1926 by Henri Almeras and launched in 1930. When Patou visited Almeras in his laboratories in Grasse in southern France, he tested numerous vials of scents and eventually settled on one containing a blend of *rose de mai* and jasmine. The perfumer told Patou that this particular perfume was far too expensive to market, but Patou took no notice and would not entertain any suggestion that the perfume should be diluted. *Joy* thus became "the costliest perfume in the world."

composing the scent

Once the fragrance oils have been chosen by the perfumer, his or her next job is to compose the scent. A perfume is "constructed" to have three movements—a beginning, middle, and end—to take account of the different evaporation rates of the oils used in a blend.

The beginning, or the top note, is your initial impression of the perfume—what you smell when you first open the bottle. The fragrances used for the top notes are usually made from fresh-smelling plants, citrus fruits, herbs, and green scents like lemons and limes, bergamot and coriander, pine and lavender. Once the perfume has been applied to the skin, the top note will begin to fade after about half an hour.

The middle of the perfume is called the heart note. It is slower to evaporate than the top note, lasting for up to four hours and thus defining the main character of the scent. The heart note—where the more precious fragrances occur—is often floral with some woody overtones. Popular fragrances for the heart note range from jasmine, rose, ylang-ylang, and orchids to lilacs, neroli, tuberose, and gardenia.

The end of the perfume is the bass note, which in turn lasts longer than both the top and heart notes. It has the slowest rate of evaporation and though it is usually apparent in the scent from the beginning, it can linger for most of the day. The bass note is also known as the dry down because the fragrances used are usually quite heavy and clingy. Bass note fragrances include musk, amber, orris, and vanilla.

All these elements are bound together by fixatives whose job it is to retard the evaporation process and in doing so blend and harmonize the scents. Without a fixative, each scent would have smelled at different rates, but a blend with too many fixatives will be flat. Balance is the key and this is where a perfumer's nose becomes critical.

fragrance families

Fragrances can be linked into family types, and the four main families are the chypres, the florals, the fougères, and the orientals. A new group, the marine or oceanic, is a recent addition to the family of fragrances.

right: **Some of the perfumes that belong to the floral group of fragrances.**

below: ***Champs-Elysées* (Guerlain) is a good example of the chypres group of scents.**

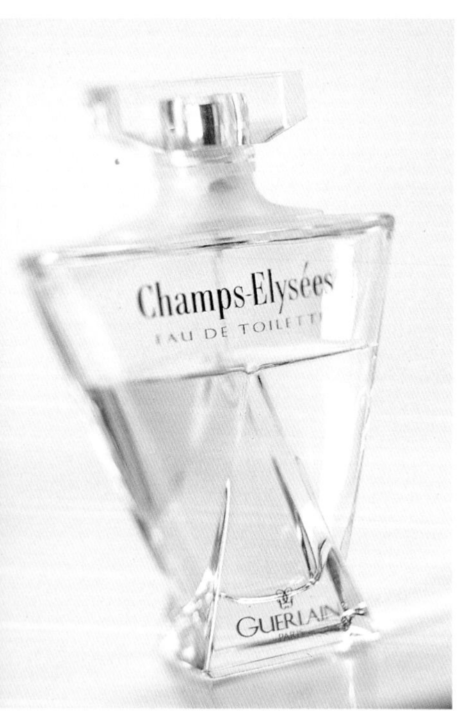

THE CHYPRES

floral chypres	— *green*
	— *fresh*
animals chypres	— *sweet*
	— *fruity*

This group of fragrances is strong, mossy, and spicy. Resins like cedarwood, and herbs like bergamot are usually used in the base note of chypre perfumes. Chypres were named after Coty's 1917 scent of the same name that combined oakmoss, orange, geranium, and spices. Within the chypre family there are two main divisions—floral and animal—and two further sub-divisions.

Floral chypres—feminine and fruity. For example *Ysatis* (Givenchy), *Paloma Picasso* (Paloma Picasso), *Y* (Yves St Laurent), and *Versace* (Versace).

Green florals—lighter than floral chypre but still quite mossy. For example *Charlie* (Revlon), *Aliage* (Estée Lauder), *Aromatics Elixir* (Clinique).

Fresh florals—herbal and uplifting. For example *CK One* (Calvin Klein), *Eau Savage* (Christian Dior), and *Fahrenheit* (Christian Dior).

Animal chypres—contain animal scents and leathery notes, making them warm and sensual. For example *Polo* (Ralph Lauren), *Jaïpur* (Boucheron), and *Jolie Madame* (Balmain).

Sweet animal chypres—intimate and erotic. For example, *Shocking* (Schiaparelli), *Intimate* (Revlon), and *Comme des Garçons* (Comme des Garçons).

Fruity animal chypres—citrus overtones. For example *Mitsouko* (Guerlain), *Montana* (Montana), and *Champagne* (Yves St Laurent).

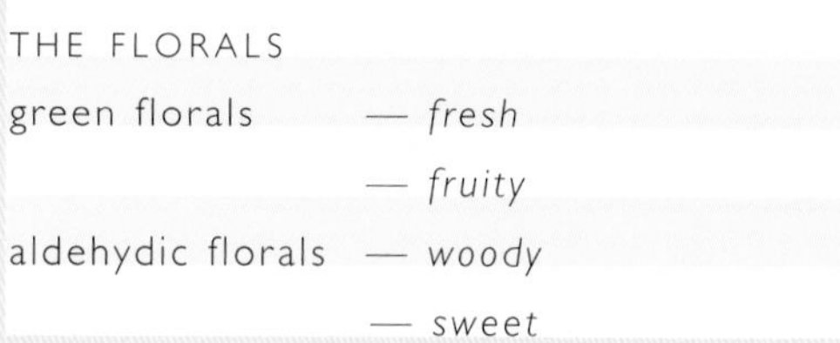

THE FLORALS

green florals	— *fresh*
	— *fruity*
aldehydic florals	— *woody*
	— *sweet*

The florals are quite simply fragrances with flowery notes. They are made by combining several flowers into a bouquet of flower notes or by using just one type to make a fragrance with a single flower note. The florals split into two categories—green and aldehydic—with two further divisions in each category.

Green florals—smell "green," redolent of freshly cut grass, leaves, light flowers, and springtime in the countryside. For example *Vert Vert* (Guerlain), *Miss Dior* (Christian Dior), *Giò* (Giorgio Armani), *Givenchy III* (Givenchy).

Fresh—crisp and effervescent fragrances. For example, *Escape* (Calvin Klein), *Sunflowers* (Elizabeth Arden), and *Safari* (Ralph Lauren).

Fruity—a combination of tangy citrus fruits and subtle florals. For example, *Anaïs Anaïs* (Cacharel), *L'eau d'Issey* (Issey Miyake), and *Trésor* (Lancôme).

Aldehydic florals—synthetic chemical combinations that highlight the depths of natural fragrances and give them a champagne-like lift. For example *Rive Gauche* (Yves St Laurent), *Madame*

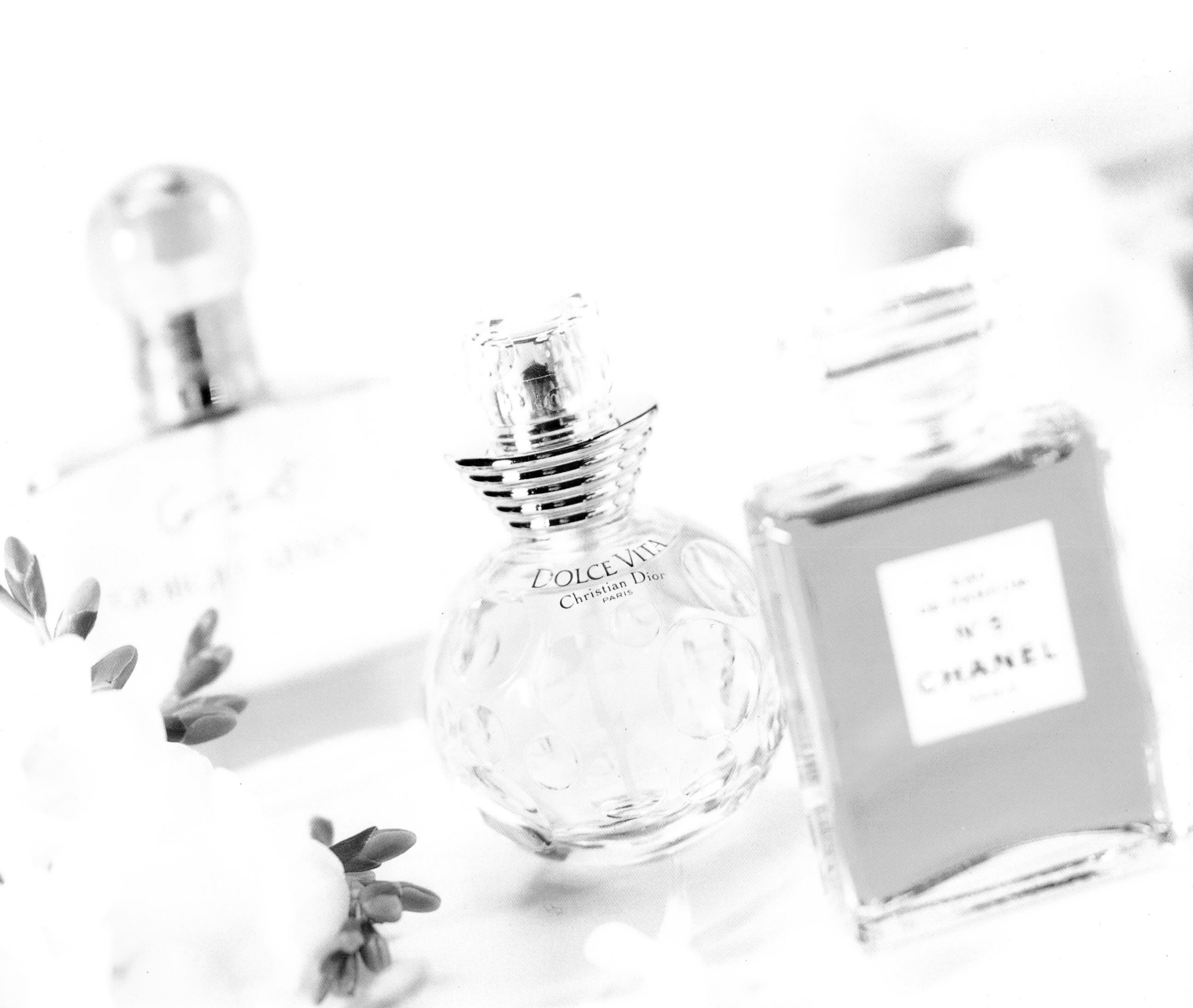
DOLCE VITA
Christian Dior
PARIS
CHANEL

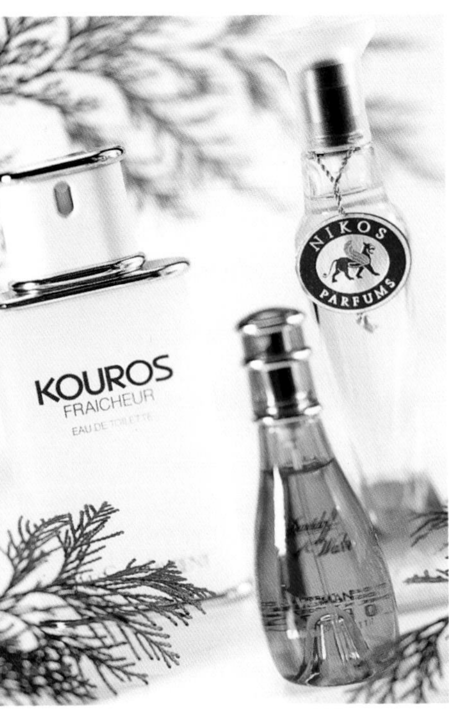

above: **A few of the perfumes which belong to the fougère family.**

Rochas (Rochas), *No. 5* (Chanel), and *First* (Van Cleef and Arpels).

Woody—have heavier notes than the previous. For example, *No. 19* (Chanel), *White Linen* (Estée Lauder), and *Dolce Vita* (Christian Dior).

Sweet—powdery and soft. For example, *L'Air du Temps* (Nina Ricci), *Blue Grass* (Elizabeth Arden), and *Beautiful* (Estée Lauder).

THE FOUGERES	
floral fougère	— *green*
	— *fresh*
leather fougère	— *spicy*
	— *woody*

Fougère means fern in French and although ferns don't actually have a scent, we imagine them to smell of woodlands and hay—fresh and aromatic. They tend to carry top notes of lavender and a base of patchouli and oakmoss. The fougères are split into two categories—floral and leather—with two divisions in each category.

Floral fougère—a distinct cooling yet quite strong aroma. For example *Wrappings* (Clinique) and *Parfum d'Eté* (Kenzo).

Green florals—lightly masculine. For example *Drakkar Noir* (Guy Laroche) and *Cool Water* (Davidoff).

Fresh florals—citrusy hints. For example *Ô de Lancôme* (Lancôme) and *English Lavender* (Yardley).

Leather fougère—more masculine overtones, being as the name suggests quite leathery with a hint of tobacco fragrance. For example *Minotaure* (Paloma Picasso) and *Brut* (Fabergé).

Spicy—a more pungent aroma. For example *Kouros* (Yves St Laurent) and *Alliage* (Estée Lauder).

Woody—a more natural fragrance. For example *Tuscany* (Aramis), and *Paco Rabanne Pour Homme* (Paco Rabanne).

THE ORIENTALS	
floral orientals	— *fruity*
	— *fruity floral*
spicy orientals	— *animal*
	— *sweet*

The oriental group of fragrances are exotic, spicy, and musky. They have intense scents that are blends of vanilla, spices, and aromatic woods. As in the other groupings, they are split into two main categories and then sub-divided again.

Floral orientals—heavy floral blend that includes a variety of spices and exotic ingredients. For example, *Shalimar* (Guerlain), *Opium* (Yves St

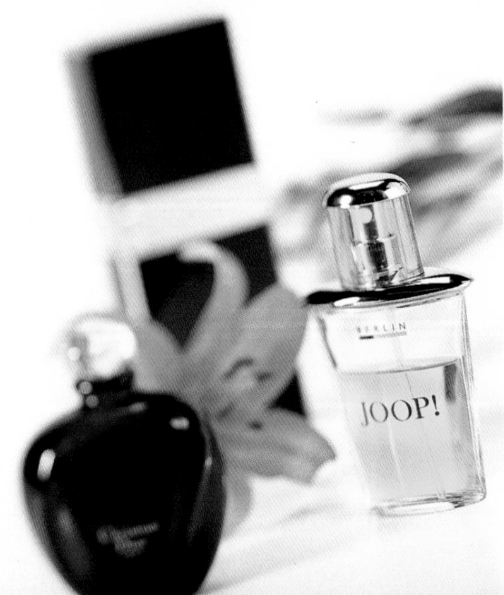

right: **Some examples of the Oriental group of fragrances.**

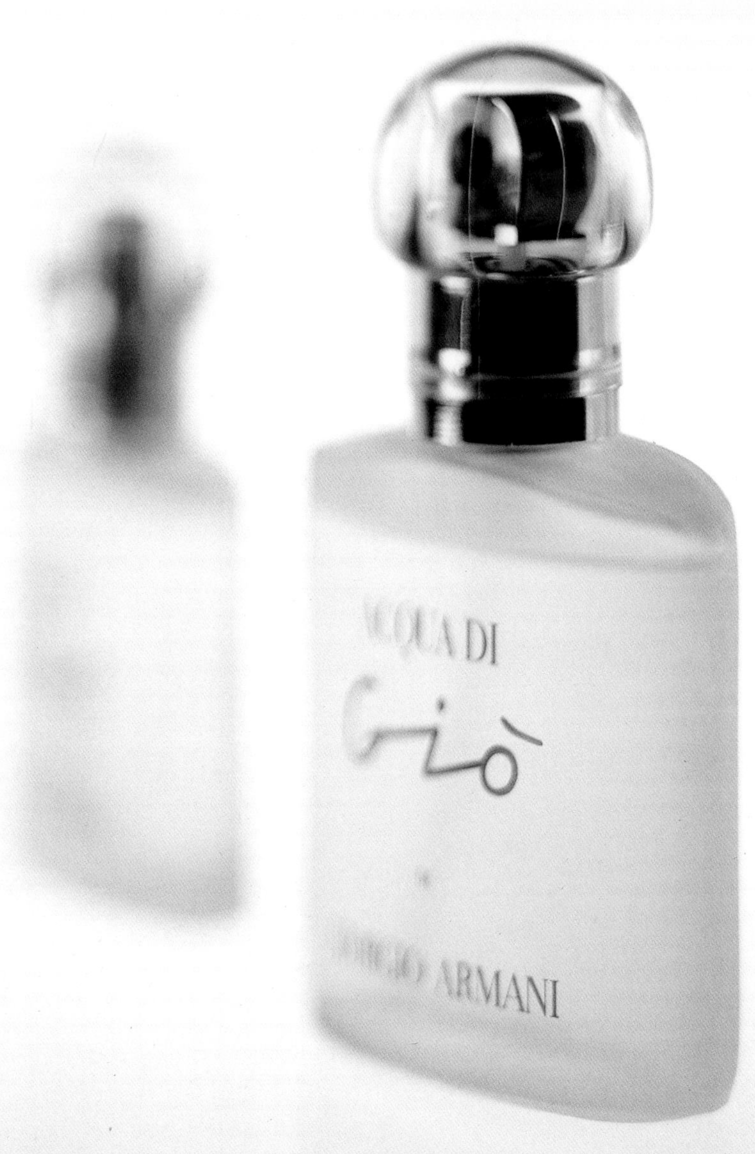

left: ***Aqua di Giò* is one of the marine group of scents.**

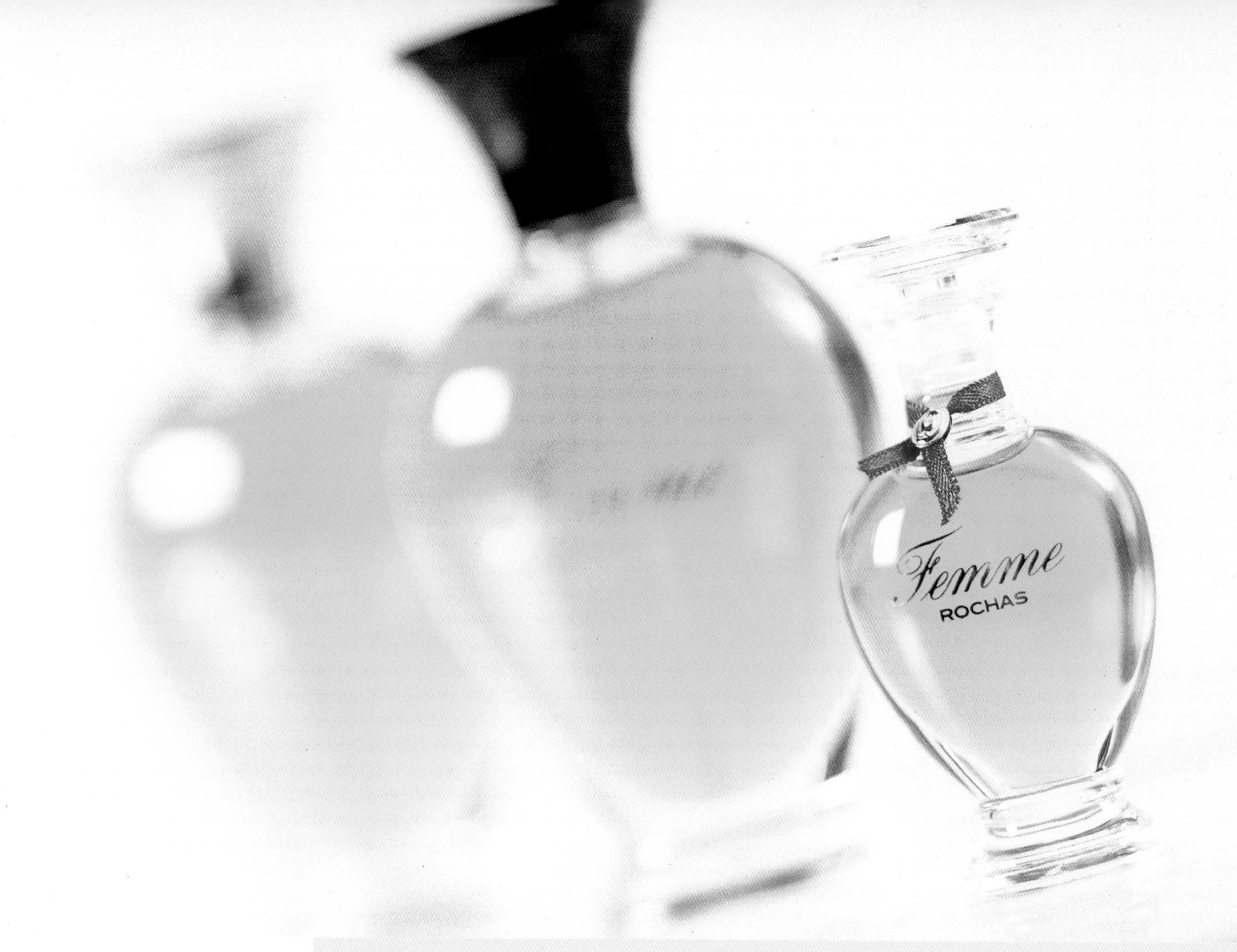

above from left: ***Femme* (Rochas) eau de toilette, eau de parfum, and pure perfume.**

Laurent), and *Panthère* (Cartier).

Fruity—touches of citrus. For example *Roma* (Laura Biagiotti), *Moschino* (Moschino), and *Sublime* (Jean Patou).

Fruity floral—for example, *Poison* (Christian Dior), *Jean Paul Gaultier* (Jean Paul Gaultier) and *Poème* (Lancôme).

Spicy orientals—aromatic spices mixed with vanilla and musks to create quite heady scents. For example *Angel* (Thierry Mugler), *Obsession* (Calvin Klein), and *Cinnabar* (Estée Lauder).

Animal—musky and amber type scents. For example, *Egoïste* (Chanel) and *Asja* (Fendi).

Sweet—more feminine and a little lighter. For example, *Donna Karan* (Donna Karan), *Must de Cartier* (Cartier), and *Amarige* (Givenchy).

MARINE OR OCEANICS

These scents are fresh, watery, and reminiscent of tangy sea air. For example, *Dune* (Christian Dior), and *Escape* (Calvin Klein).

degrees of perfume

Extrait—a pure perfume with the highest concentration of fragrance oils in alcohol. Concentration of 15 to 40 percent.

Eau de parfum—a blend of fragrance oils mixed with distilled water and alcohol. Concentration of 10 to 20 percent.

Eau de toilette—a blend of the oils, water, and alcohol but at a lower concentration. A perfumer will often change the balance of a perfume, from the *extrait* to the eau de toilette, so that it has fresher top notes. Concentration of 8 to 10 percent.

Eau de Cologne/Eau Fraîche—an even softer blend of oils, water, and alcohol. Concentration of 3 to 5 percent.

Most modern perfumes have further additives, like sunscreens and preservatives, that can alter the final smell of the perfume.

Mood-altering perfumes

Scientific research has proven that smells stimulate the brain, releasing chemicals that are capable of a vast range of functions. Retailers have grown wise to the way that fragrances can make one feel, so much so that they use smells to influence our spending habits and our lives—and they do it without us even noticing. Supermarkets permeate their bakery stands with synthetic smells of freshly baked bread, and in Japan fragrances are filtered through the air-conditioning systems to encourage the workforce to be more productive.

Scents can conjure childhood memories and instill certain feelings. It is as though we can be unconsciously conditioned by the mere whiff of some nostalgic fragrance. This notion attracted not only the attention of the perfume manufacturers but also of the medical professional. "Odor conditioning" is fast becoming a retail and medical term to describe how smells are used to condition us to spend, spend, spend or to lead healthier and more harmonious lives. Clinique's *Happy* includes five newly created synthetic fragrance notes that, according to the market research carried out prior to launch, each have a revitalizing effect on the wearer and anyone who inhales the scent. Manufacturers The Gap and Aveda have been using the pioneering methods of "mind wardrobes." These fragrances apparently contain mood essences, which is why Aveda named their scents *Motivation*, *Attraction*, and *Intuition*. The Gap has opted for more evocative names like *Earth* and *Heaven*.

Many fragrances are said to be able to affect your frame of mind and to enhance certain moods. The following chart shows you which fragrances and perfumes can affect your mood or fulfil certain needs.

mood	fragrance	perfumes
To boost energy levels and overcome feelings of apathy.	Cool and refreshing scents that contain the essential oils of peppermint, eucalyptus, rosemary, and grapefruit are ideal. Avoid warm perfumes and stick to the uplifting aromas.	*CK One* (Calvin Klein) *L'eau d'Issey* (Issey Miyake) *Paco* (Paco Rabanne) *Ice* (Byblos)
To overcome insecurity and hypersensitivity, and to boost self-confidence.	Soft florals with essences of geranium, chamomile, and rose.	*Envy* (Gucci) *True Love* (Elizabeth Arden) *Pleasures* (Estée Lauder) *Byzantine* (Rochas)
To improve work performance and increase assertiveness.	Fresh, herbal scents with essences of cedarwood, basil, bergamot, and lemon.	*Miss Dior* (Christian Dior) *Versace* (Versace) *Aliage* (Estée Lauder) *Y* (Yves St Laurent)
To unwind and escape reality.	Orientals, spices, and woods, like cedarwood, frankincense, sage, and ylang-ylang.	*Coco* (Chanel) *Obsession* (Calvin Klein) *Opium* (Yves St Laurent) *Amarige* (Givenchy)
To enhance femininity and heighten sexual awareness.	Floral Oriental fragrances, like jasmine, tuberose, and those containing aldehydes.	*First* (Van Cleef and Arpels) *Chloe Narcisse* (Chloe) *So de la Renta* (Oscar de la Renta) *Rive Gauche* (Yves St Laurent)
To heighten self-expression and imbue a sense of freedom.	Fruit and food smells, like grapefruit and pimento.	*Angel* (Thierry Mugler) *Sun, Moon, Stars* (Karl Lagerfeld) *Tiffany* (Tiffany) *Casmir* (Chopan)

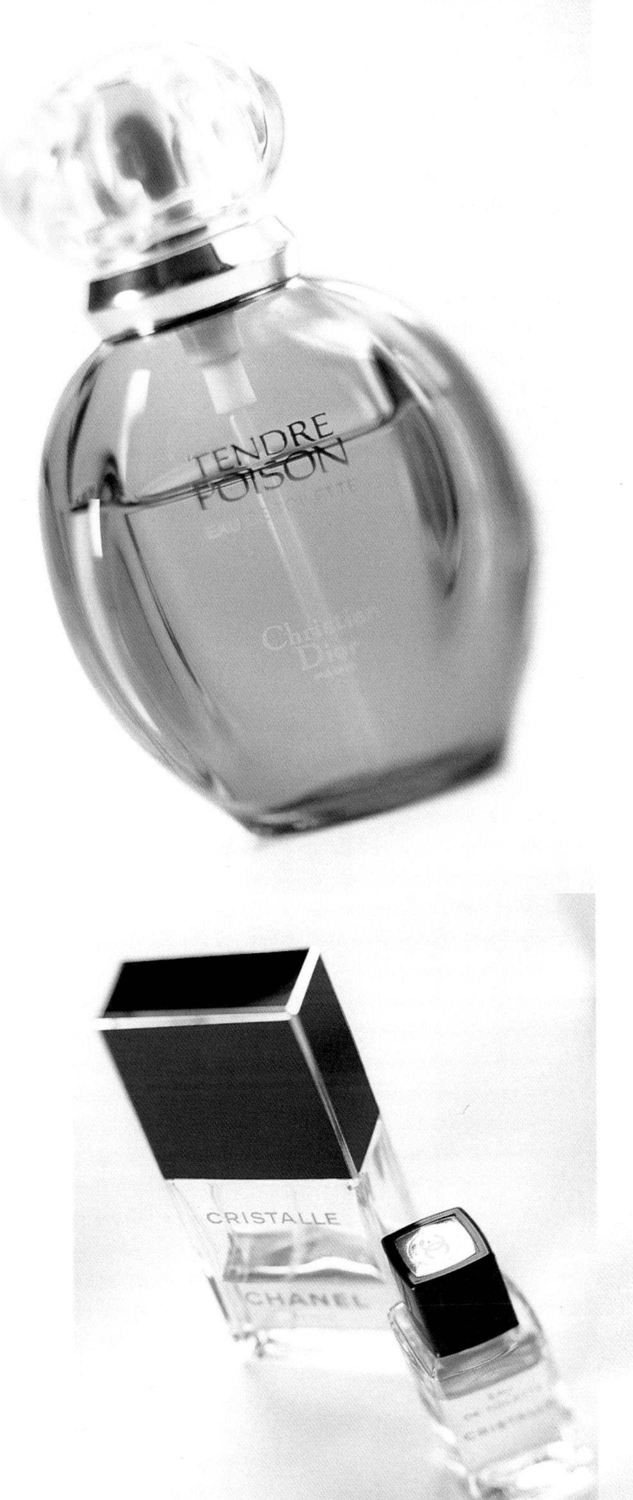
TENDRE POISON
Christian Dior
CRISTALLE
CHANEL

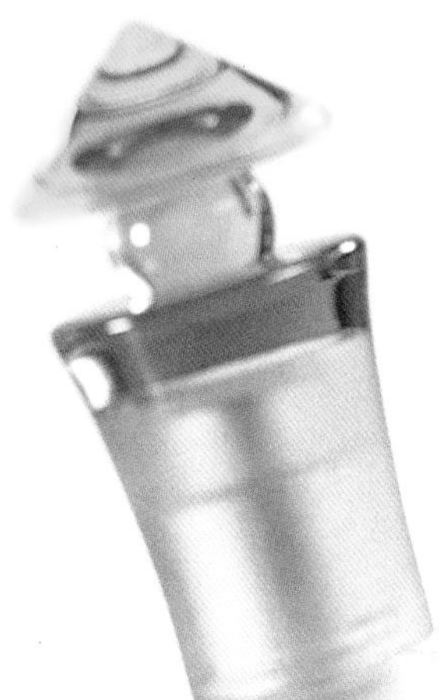

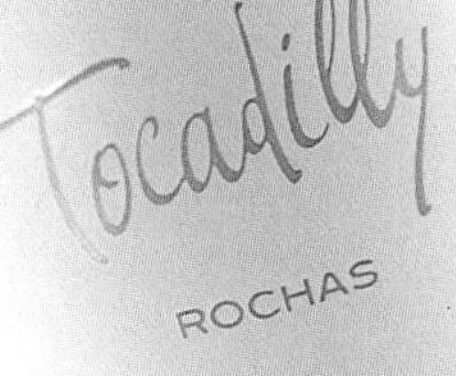
Tocadilly
ROCHAS

chapter 3

essentia and arom

l oils
atherapy

WHAT ARE ESSENTIAL OILS?

Our sense of smell is one of our most powerful senses, therefore smells that we find attractive and appealing will positively affect the way we feel physically and emotionally. From this we must also accept that unpleasant smells will have a negative effect.

Just as the smell of vanilla ice cream can evoke happy memories of a long-forgotten childhood summer vacation, and pine cones of Yuletide festivities, essential oils can foster and heighten feelings of comfort and good health. It is these essential oils that are used in the practice of aromatherapy.

Essential oils are the concentrated essences derived from flowers, fruit, leaves, seeds, and bark by steam distillation. Often the essential oil is so highly concentrated that many plants are used to produce just a tiny amount of oil. It takes more than two dozen roses to produce a single drop of rose essential oil. When a number of oils are used in combination they can reputedly promote physical and emotional well-being on a number of levels.

Different essential oils have different qualities as illustrated in the charts that follow. Frankincense clears the mind, and eucalyptus purifies the atmosphere, which is why it is planted in marsh lands to prevent malaria. There is a wonderful tale that tells how the soldiers of ancient Greece were forbidden peppermint in times of war because it was common knowledge that peppermint had aphrodisiac qualities!

Aromatherapy is concerned with discovering and utilizing the beneficial effects of essential oils to aid physical and emotional healing and to enhance personal vitality and spirituality. To effect these benefits, aromatherapy employs not only our sense of smell but also our wonderful sense of touch. Oils can be added to a bath so that we inhale their fragrance, or massaged into the skin to relieve stress and anxiety, aches and pains, as well as conditions such as depression and skin problems. In both instances, inhalation and touch work together. An aromatherapy bath, for example, lets you inhale the aroma while your body is comforted by the warm fragranced water and relaxing surroundings.

history of aromatherapy

Aromatherapy has been in practice throughout the world for thousands of years. It has developed from ancient times when natural fragrances and incense were burned in the temples of the Egyptians with the aim of creating an atmosphere of mental restoration and calm. Such an atmosphere was conducive to the worshipping of their various deities.

As far back as 3500 BC the temples of Egypt were burning resins like frankincense and cedarwood to clear the mind and encourage meditation. According to legend, sandalwood was used in the temples of Solomon to "perfume the devotions of his worshippers" and its reputed benefits include tranquility, wisdom, and sensitivity.

It was only in 1937 that aromatherapy was given its name by a French chemist called René-Maurice Gatefousse. Gatefousse worked with essential oils in a perfume laboratory and, after burning his hand quite badly, he plunged it into the bowl of liquid beside him—a bowl containing pure lavender essential oil. His noticed that his hand healed very quickly with minimal scarring and so began his research into essential oils. His exhaustive research led him to discover that many essential oils had healing and antiseptic qualities.

Throughout the Second World War, another Frenchman, Dr. Jean Valnet, added to Gatefousse's research. But, unlike Gatefousse who worked in the sterile surroundings of a laboratory, Valnet did his practical research while a field surgeon. In part, Valnet's research into essential oils was prompted by a dire shortage of traditional medical supplies. His experience also confirmed that essential oils were successful in aiding healing.

Many people are skeptical about aromatherapy. They draw attention to the distinct lack of scientific research to support years of anecdotal evidence. But in spite of this, aromatherapy is the fastest-growing complementary therapy in the United States, Europe, Australia, and the United Kingdom, with more and more health professionals using it in their practices.

Some health professionals insist that the concept of aromatherapy is not so different from traditional medical practices. Many pharmaceutical drugs have a base of natural oils to which other compounds are added. All aromatherapy does is remove the chemical element to ensure a purely natural remedy. As more research is being undertaken, evidence tends to favor aromatherapy. The few group studies that have been done attest to the fact that patients who may not physically benefit from aromatherapy massages are definitely benefiting psychologically.

how essential oil aromas affect us

It is reputed that the aromas of the essential oils affect us in three distinct ways.

*When certain oils are inhaled they are thought to stimulate the olfactory nerve that in turn

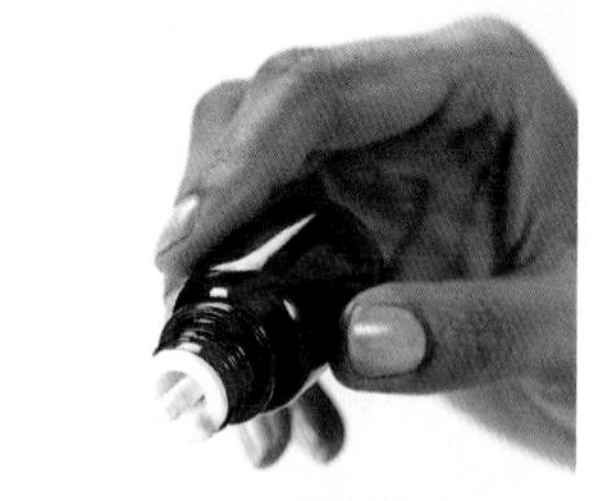
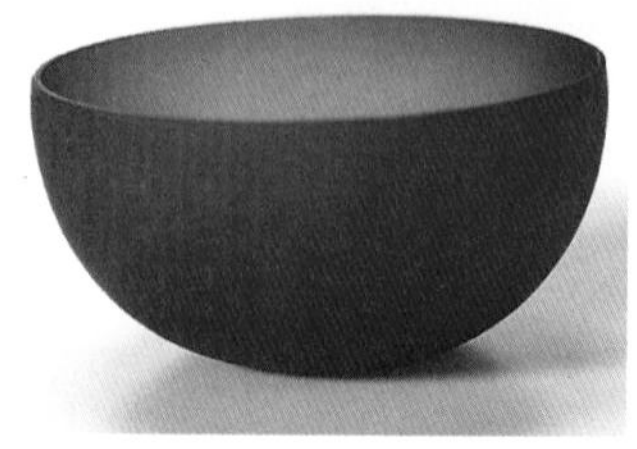

above: **Adding essential oil to base oil for massage.**

affects the limbic system. The limbic system is that part of the brain that governs memory, intuition, and emotional aspects of our behavior. Carefully chosen oils can apparently influence this system and thus have some effect upon any disorders. Basil and rosemary, for example, are said to improve memory, while frankincense and sandalwood enhance intuition.

*The aroma of the essential oils passes through the limbic system to the hypothalamus. The hypothalamus governs the pituitary gland and regulates endocrine activity, controlling the hormonal system, and our glands. The odor of certain essential oils can encourage the release of neurochemicals like dopamine and serotonin. Dopamine instills feelings of well-being, and serotonin has sedative effects.

*Some essential oils have a very tiny molecular structure that can permeate the skin cells and enter the bloodstream when massaged into the skin with a base or carrier oil. Once absorbed into the skin some essential oils can relieve tension and anxiety, although this has yet to be medically proven.

It must be remembered that the aroma of essential oils has been appreciated for centuries in its own right. The refreshing and stimulating scent of eucalyptus has been used for centuries to provide relief from congestion. Sweet-smelling orange and clove pomanders were used in seventeenth century Europe to combat the stench of rotting bodies during the Black Death, and to ward off this plague, the latter use being based more in superstition than in fact.

methods of using essential oils

Massage

This is believed to be the most effective way to use essential oils in aromatherapy. The essential oil should be combined with a base oil, or carrier oil. Vegetable oils are best for this purpose, and those with a minimal fragrance such as almond or sunflower oil are ideal. A basic blend should be 3 drops of essential oil to 1 teaspoon of base oil.

Massaging the feet and hands is a great way to keep in good health as it stimulates the reflex points for the body. But before carrying out a full-body massage with essential oils it is advised that you should take a course in aromatherapy massage.

Bathing

This is an easy and highly enjoyable way to use essential oils. Run a bath with warm water—hot water will cause the oils to dissolve too rapidly. Add an essential oil to the bath in these quantities: 5 drops of pure essential oil or 1 teaspoon of a blended essential oil and base oil (as described above). Agitate the water to blend the oils,

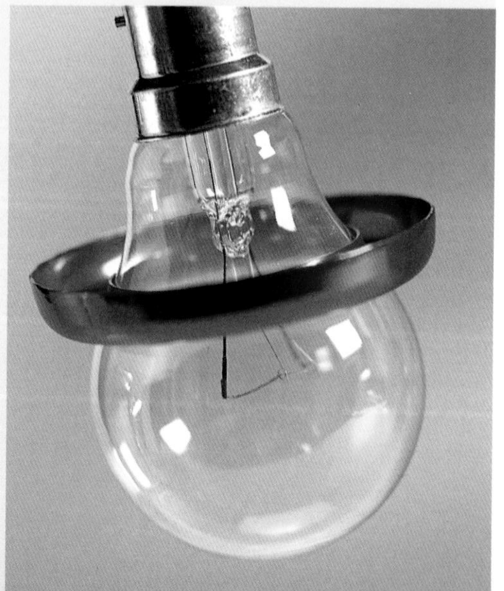

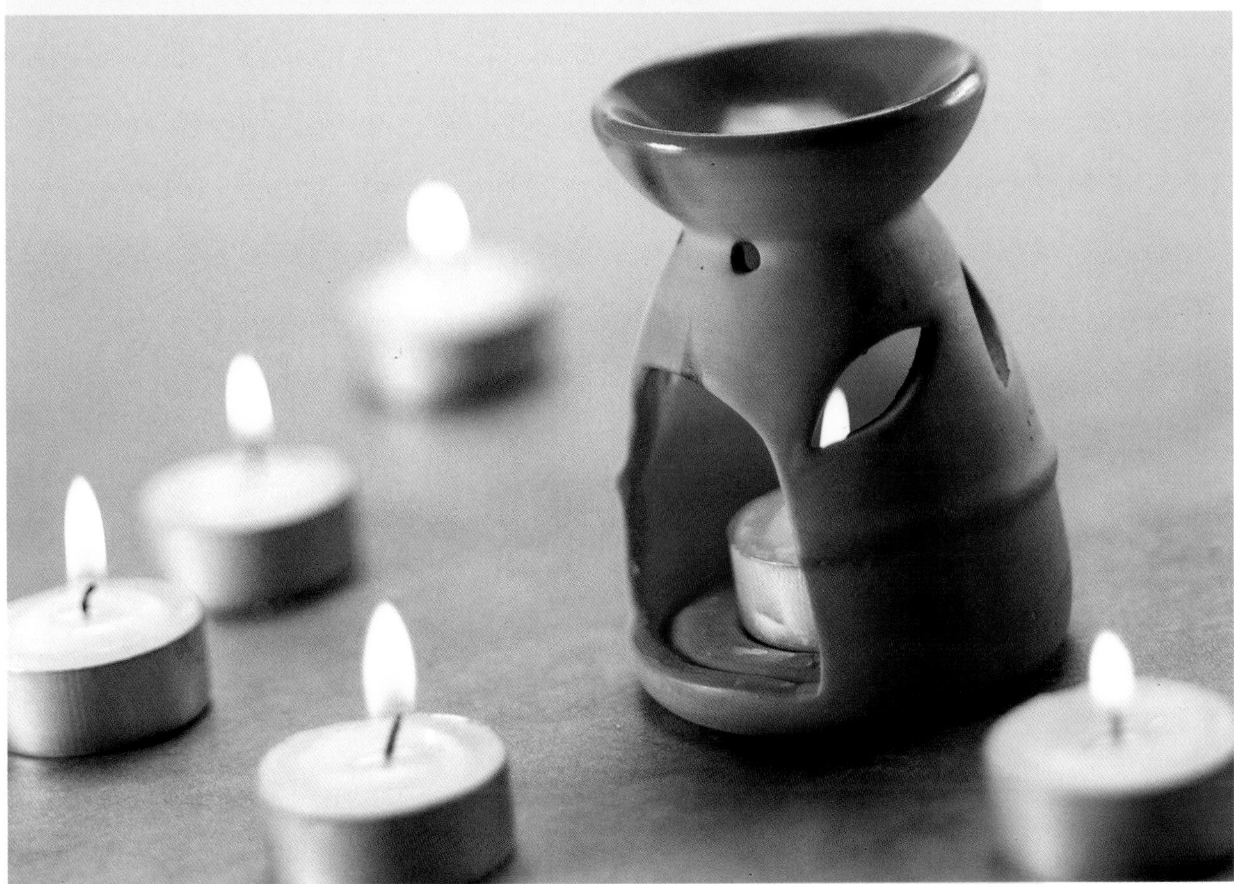

above: **Terracotta or clay burners are a popular way of using essential oils.**

then relax in the bath for at least 15 minutes.

Room fragrances

An essential oil burner is probably the most popular way of using essential oils in the home. Burners are usually made of terracotta or clay, with a recessed reservoir at the top and a space for a night light candle below. Fill the reservoir with water and then add up to 5 drops of essential oil. As the candle burns, it gently heats the reservoir and the aroma of the essential oil evaporates and is released into the air. Specific oils can be used to enhance particular moods. Lavender is ideal for creating a soothing and relaxed atmosphere, and rose wood for settling tired and grumpy older children.

A neat and safe way to use essential oils in the presence of children is to put a couple of drops of oil onto a cold light bulb, or into a ceramic ring that fits around the bulb. When the light is switched on and the bulb warms, it heats up the oil and the fragrance will gradually permeate the room. More ideas for scenting your environment are given in chapter 6, The Aromatic Home.

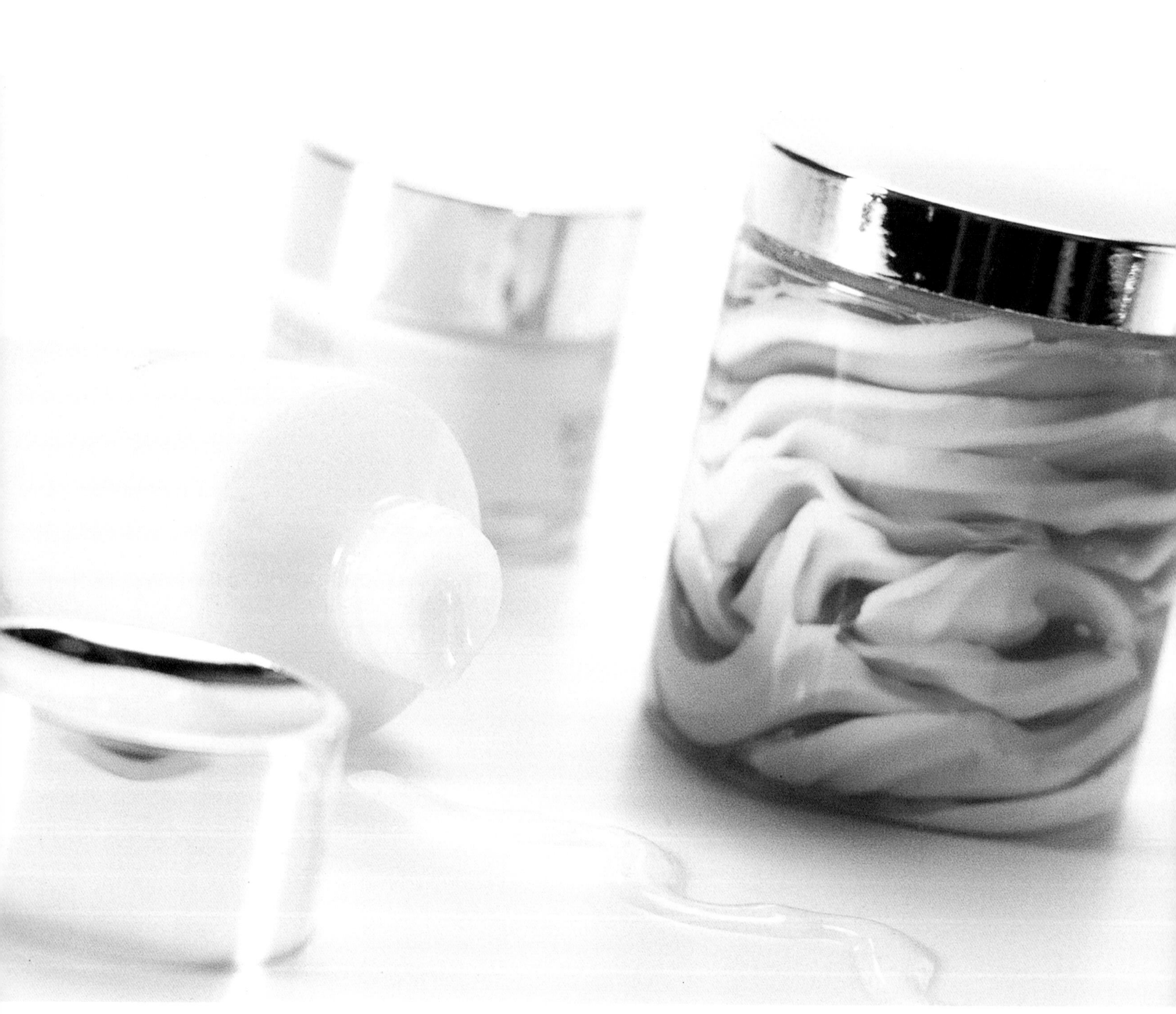

Creams, lotions, and perfumes

Face, hand, and body creams and lotions can be made by adding a few drops of essential oil to an uncolored and unscented cream. The essential oils perfume the cream and also provide soothing elements. Some essential oils are not suitable for those with sensitive skins, and a list of of these can be found later in this chapter. Recipes to make your own creams, bath oils, lip balm, and skin toners can be found in chapter 5, Fragrant Pampering.

Vaporization and inhalation

An ideal method for treating respiratory tract problems is to fill a washbowl with boiling water and then add a few drops of an appropriate essential oil. Put a towel over your head, close your eyes, and inhale the vapors for as long as it is comfortable. When traveling or working, place one or two drops of an essential oil onto a handkerchief or tissue. Put the handkerchief near, but not in contact with, your nose when you want to inhale the scent. Do not let the handkerchief go near your eyes.

using essential oils safely

For children under seven—use only lavender or Roman chamomile in a room fragrancer, or 1 or 2 drops diluted in 3 teaspoons of almond oil for a hand or foot massage.

For children between seven and 12, and pregnant women—only use half the amount of essential oil recommended for adults. The quantity of the diluting base oil remains the same.

Pregnant women—seek professional advice before using any essential oil, and the following oils should not be used: basil, clove, cinnamon, fennel, hyssop, juniper, marjoram, myrrh, peppermint, rosemary, sage, and thyme. These oils are either too stimulating or have an emmenagogic effect which will bring on menstrual periods.

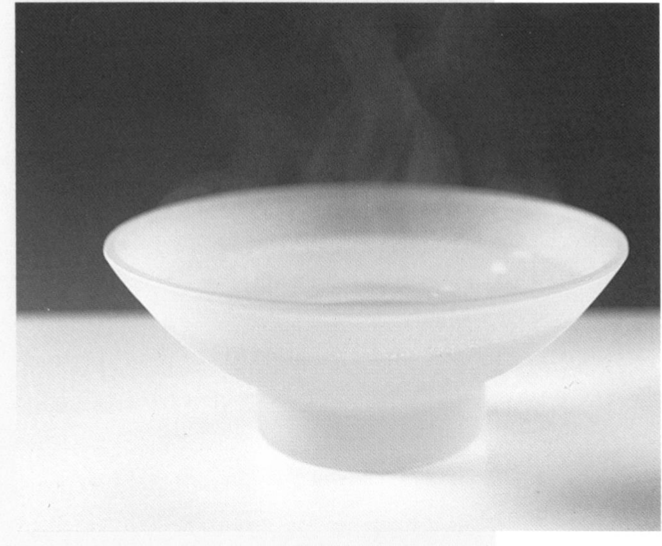

above: **Steam inhalation can help clear congested nasal passages.**

General safety

1. Never apply undiluted essential oil directly on the skin or take it internally. Keep oils away from the eyes. If an accident does occur, apply a base oil to the area to dilute the essential oil and then wash the area with plenty of water. ESSENTIAL OILS SHOULD NEVER BE TAKEN INTERNALLY.

2. If you are receiving homeopathic treatment, consult your homeopath before you receive any aromatherapy treatment.

3. If a skin irritation occurs as a reaction to an essential oil, massage almond oil into the affected area. The irritation should disappear within an hour.

ESSENTIAL OILS AND THEIR PROPERTIES

basil

Fragrance—derived from the culinary herb, which has a light, fresh, and slightly peppery fragrance.

Properties—invigorates and clears the mind giving heightened clarity, making it ideal to use during examination periods. It should be used in very small quantities and mixes well with geranium and citrus essential oils.

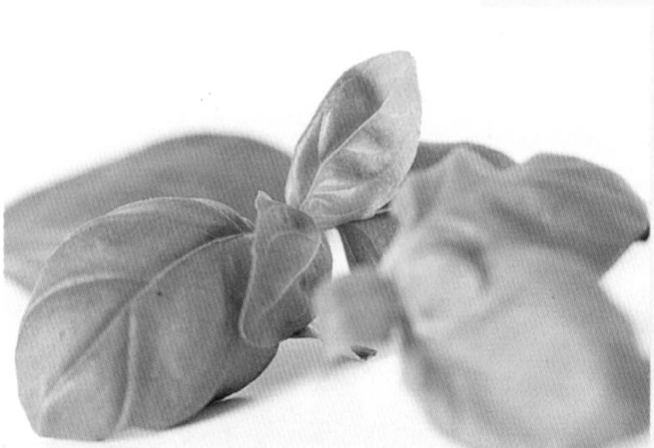

Beneficial for—improves concentration and poor memory, and encourages mental stimulation. Also good for correcting oily skin.

Safety—not suitable for children or for those with sensitive skin. Do not use during pregnancy.

Usage—for bathing, vaporization, and as insect repellent.

above: **Basil.**

right: **Chamomile.**

bergamot

Fragrance—obtained from a small orange-like fruit that is native to Italy. It has an uplifting, light citrus aroma with a very refreshing edge.

Properties—invigorating, especially in hot weather. It has a dual action, which sedates then uplifts, relaxes then refreshes. Bergamot apparently sharpens and revitalizes and is especially good for controlling eating patterns. It blends well with other oils.

Beneficial for—countering anxiety, depression, regret, stress, apathy, and lack of confidence. It can also help acne sufferers.

Safety—do not use on children or in strong sunlight.

Usage—for bathing, massage, vaporization, skin care, and as an insect repellent.

cedarwood

Fragrance—pleasant, woody, and smoky odor.

Properties—it is an astringent, and when inhaled has a composing and comforting effect. It is ideal for easing catarrh and colds.

Beneficial for—soothing a stressful and restless mind. It is also good for protecting the skin and for correcting oily skin.

Safety—do not use during pregnancy.

Usage—for bathing, massage, vaporization, skin care, and as an insect repellent.

chamomile roman

Fragrance—strong and soothing with a distinctive aroma due to its containing aculene.

Properties—very soothing and gentle oil that

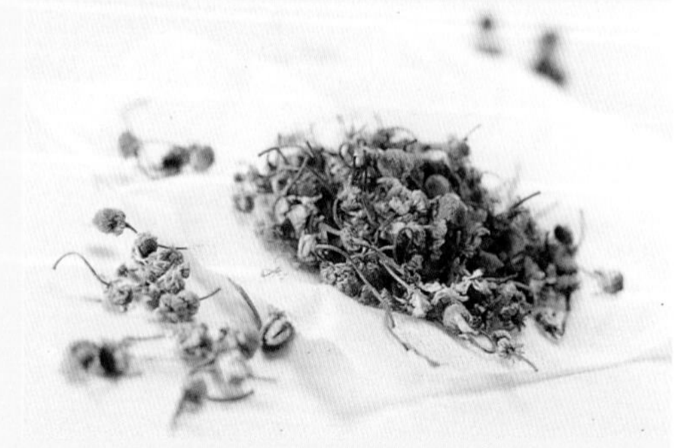

makes it suitable for young and old alike. It is excellent for dry skin as it has anti-inflammatory qualities. It will also comfort those who suffer allergies during periods of high pollen count.

Beneficial for—impulsiveness, excessive worry, irritability, and restlessness.

Safety—suitable for use with most people.

Usage—for bathing, massage, vaporization, and skin care.

cinnamon

Fragrance—distinctive warm and spicy aroma.

Properties—used traditionally for digestive problems, but it also has antiseptic qualities.

Beneficial for—easing many kinds of fever.

Safety—do not use on sensitive skins or during pregnancy.

Usage—for vaporization and as a disinfectant.

clary sage

Fragrance—the oil is steam-distilled from the entire plant and has a particularly nutty, warm, and sensual scent.

Properties—it can be soothing and relaxing, while at the same time being uplifting and encouraging feelings of well-being. It is a muscle relaxant and is apparently good to counter premenstrual tension.

Beneficial for—depression, insomnia, stress, claustrophobia, and exhaustion.

Safety—do not use during pregnancy, nor in conjunction with alcohol as it is quite euphoric.

Usage—for bathing, massage, and vaporization.

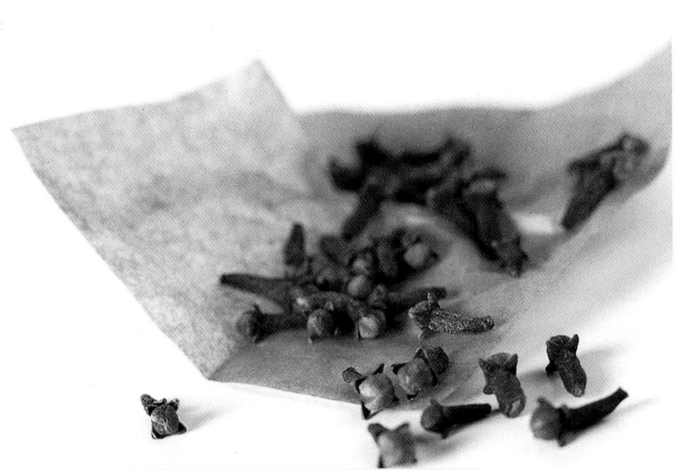

above: **Cloves.**

clove

Fragrance—made from the flower buds of small evergreen trees in Madagascar.

Properties—it is an antiseptic that is used traditionally to relieve the pain of toothache.

Beneficial for—mouth and teeth problems.

Safety—do not use on sensitive skins or during pregnancy.

Usage—vaporization and as a disinfectant.

eucalyptus

Fragrance—aromatic, sweet aroma.

Properties—Has antiseptic qualities, and is ideal to use in an essential oil burner in a sick room.

Beneficial for—the respiratory system as it is very stimulating and cleansing.

Safety—not suitable for children or those with sensitive skins, or when taking part in homeopathic treatment.

Usage—inhalant, vaporization, and as a chest rub.

below: **Eucalyptus.**

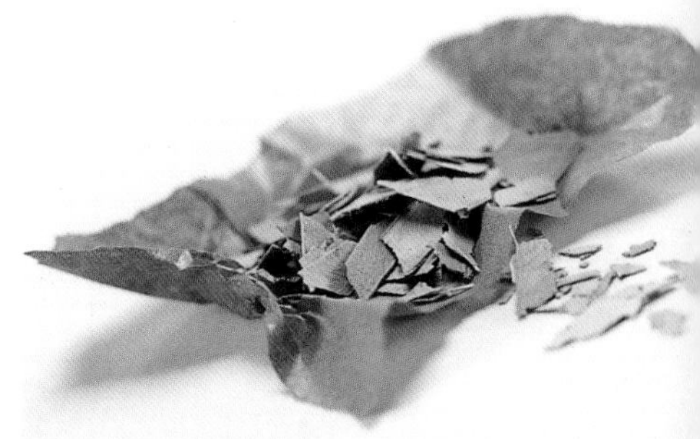

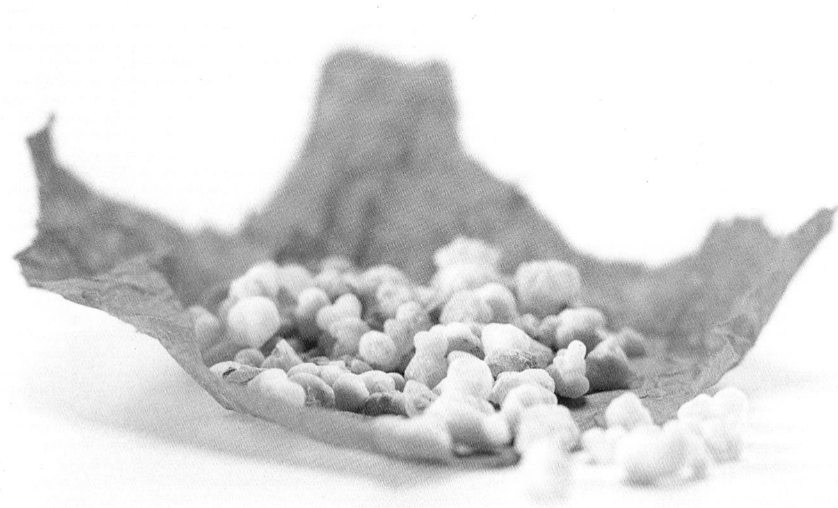

above: **Frankincense.**

below right: **Ginger.**

frankincense

Fragrance—distilled from the gum of a small North African tree, it has a warm and spicy fragrance that is historically acknowledged to be both mystical and enchanting.

Properties—soothing and meditative, helping to slow rapid breathing. Good to use on mature skin.

Beneficial for—promoting feelings of security and for relieving paranoia and fear. During a bereavement, it is comforting and warming.

Safety—not suitable for children.

Usage—for bathing, massage, vaporization, and skin care.

geranium

Fragrance—distilled from the flower of the rose geranium that is native to Madagascar. It has a fresh, sweet, floral aroma.

Properties—it has astringent qualities, making it stimulating to the lymphatic system. It also has a balancing effect which harmonizes mind and body.

Beneficial for—restoring and maintaining the stability of emotions, to correct mood swings, and rigidity. Also used in massage for lessening the appearance of cellulite.

Safety—do not use during pregnancy.

Usage—for bathing, massage, vaporization, skin care, and as a disinfectant.

ginger

Fragrance—strong, warm, and spicy aroma.

Properties—it is a warming oil, so is especially good to use in winter, and is an ideal treatment for lethargy. It is quite strong, so only use in very small quantities.

Beneficial for—increasing self-awareness and acceptance, and as a muscle relaxant. It is both fortifying and fiery, blending well with lighter oils, especially orange.

Safety—do not use on sensitive skin.

Usage—for bathing, massage, and vaporization.

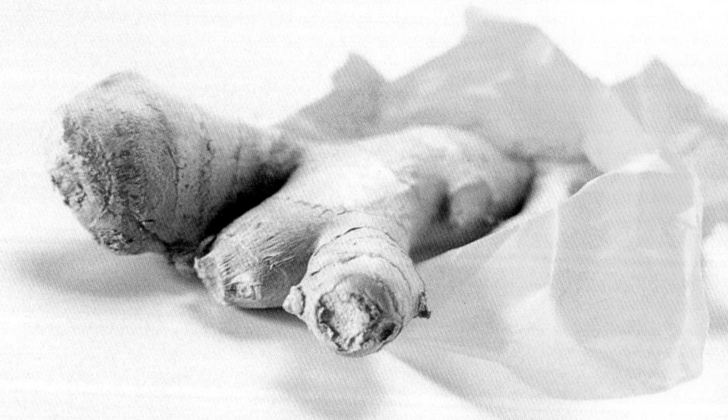

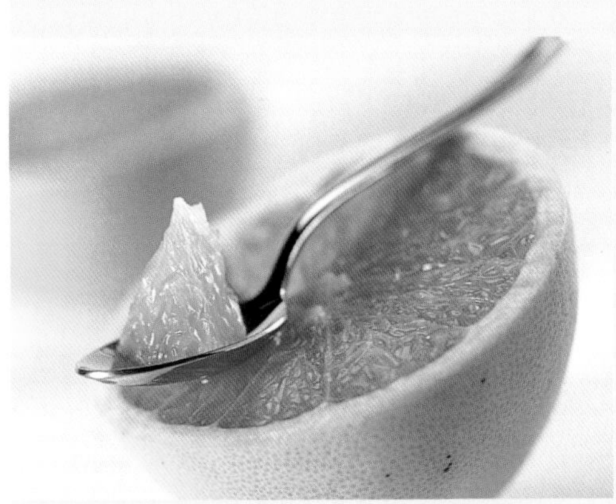

grapefruit

Fragrance—tangy, uplifting, and fresh scent.

Properties—reviving quality for the spirit, while also being relaxing and balancing. It encourages a regular appetite as it is good for the digestive system. It may aid overcoming jetlag, and is reputedly beneficial for indecisiveness, confusion, frustration, and envy. It can foster clarity of thought and action.

Safety—do not use in strong sunlight.

Usage—for bathing, massage, and vaporization.

jasmine

Fragrance—referred to as the king of all the flower oils, it is the most expensive oil and has a luxurious, exotic perfume. Kama, the Hindu god of love, has been pictured with jasmine blossoms on the end of his arrows—the aphrodisiac qualities of jasmine will supposedly pierce the heart with desire.

Properties—eases depression and calms anxiety. It is known for its aphrodisiac qualities as well as being a good skin care oil.

Beneficial for—apathy, fear, rigidity, and sadness, as it is relaxing and emotionally warming.

Safety—do not use on sensitive skins or during pregnancy.

Usage—for bathing, massage, vaporization, and skin-care.

juniper

Fragrance—invigorating and woody.

Properties—it has cleansing, antiseptic, and astringent properties and is known to be blood purifying.

Beneficial for—countering lethargy and it is seen to be protective and purifying.

Safety—do not use during pregnancy.

Usage—for bathing, massage, vaporization, and as a disinfectant.

lavender

Fragrance—possibly the best-known and most widely used essential oil with a fresh and sweet fragrance.

Properties—it is a versatile oil being refreshing for

above left: **Grapefruit.**

below: **Lavender.**

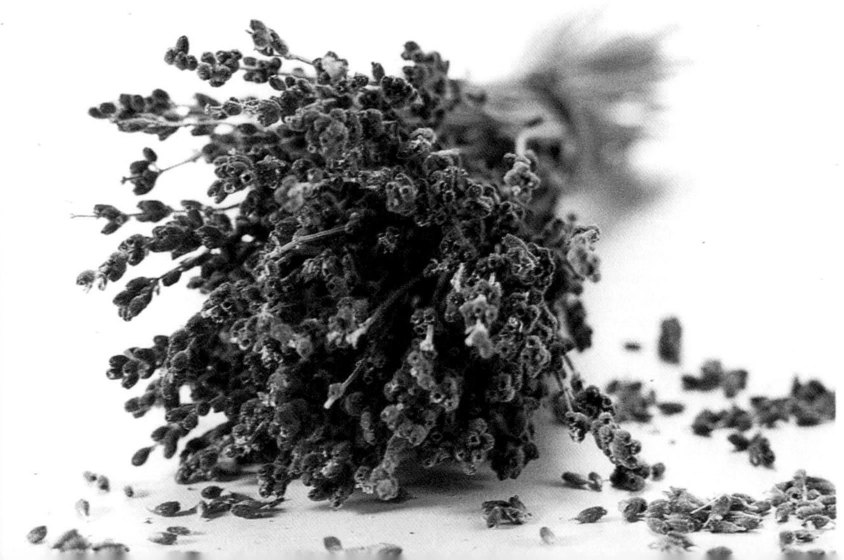

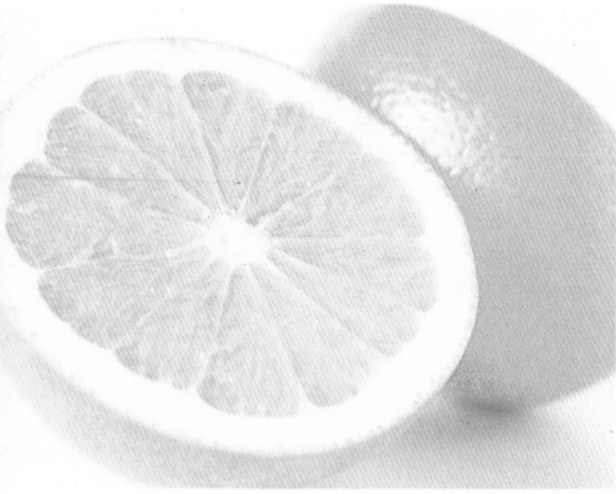

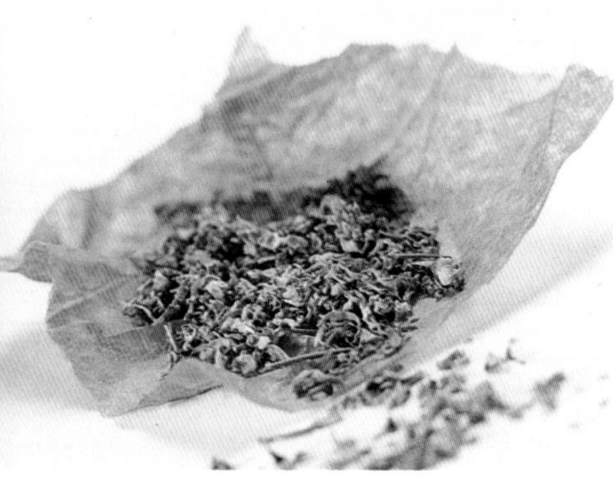

top: **Lemon.**

above: **Marjoram.**

right: **Myrrh.**

tired muscles and extremely good to use in the winter. One or two drops on your pillow at night will aid restful sleep.

Beneficial for—quelling fear, impatience, insomnia, restlessness, and anxiety. It will also restore equilibrium.

Safety—suitable for most people, even young children.

Usage—for bathing, massage, vaporization, skin care, foot baths, and as a disinfectant and insect repellent.

lemon

Fragrance—made from the rind of the fruit, it takes about three thousand lemons to produce just two pounds of the essential oil. It has a refreshing, tangy aroma.

Properties—good medicine for warts and verrucas, and it also stems the blood flow from wounds and benefits blood circulation.

Beneficial for—countering sluggishness as it encourages brightness, mental clarity, and focus. It is a refreshing tonic that cools and stimulates.

Safety—do not use on sensitive skin or in direct sunlight.

Usage—for bathing, massage, vaporization, and as a disinfectant.

marjoram

Fragrance—warming and soothing.

Properties—can provide relief from tired muscles and menstrual discomfort. It is also an aid to peaceful sleep.

Beneficial for—countering fatigue, mental strain, grief, and loneliness. It is an ideal relaxant.

Safety—do not use during pregnancy.

Usage—for bathing, massage, and vaporization.

melissa (lemon balm)

Fragrance—sweet and lemony.

Properties—it is both soothing and uplifting for the mind and body, and provides comfort for those with nervous dispositions and colds.

Beneficial for—sedating and as a gentle tonic for worry and shock. It has been called the "elixir for life" and can help those with allergies.

Safety—do not use during pregnancy and on sensitive skin.

Usage—for bathing, massage, vaporization, and as an insect repellent.

myrrh

Fragrance—one of the oldest essential oils, having a deep religious significance along with frankincense. It has a smoky and mysterious scent.

Properties—ideal to use as a wash or gargle for mouth and throat infections. Can also be added to creams for the prevention of chapped skin.

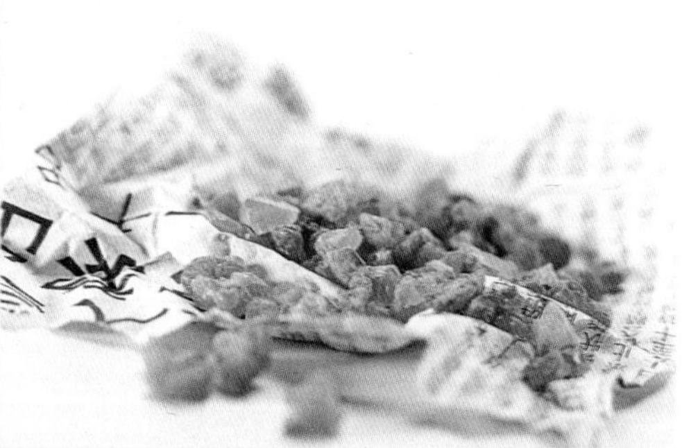

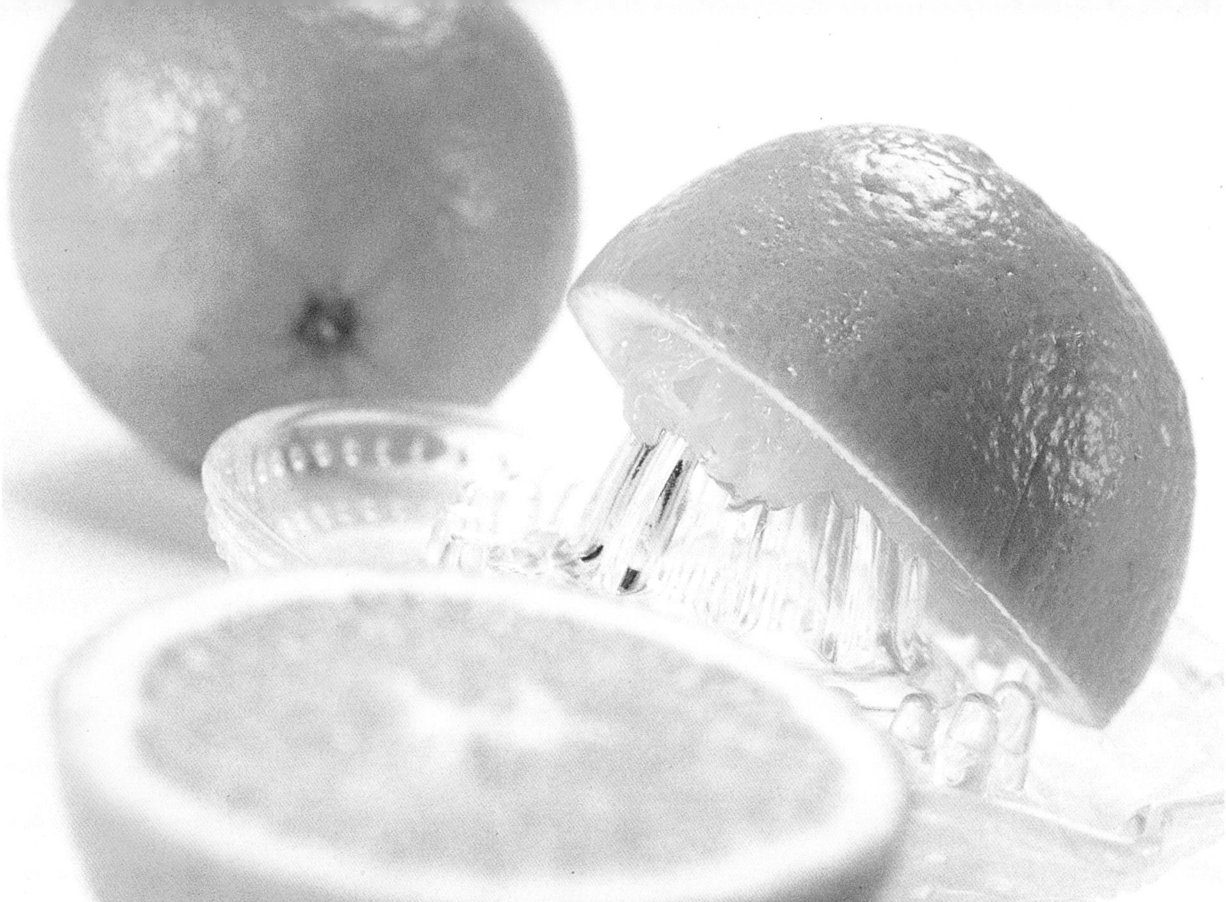

above: **Orange.**

Beneficial for—countering body odor.

Safety—do not use on sensitive skin or during pregnancy.

Usage—for bathing, massage, vaporization, and as an insect repellent.

orange

Fragrance—sweet and radiant.

Properties—known as a warm and cheering oil, it is good for those who lack energy.

Beneficial for—the digestive system and when one is feeling low. It blends especially well with spice oils for winter baths.

Safety—do not use during pregnancy.

Usage—for bathing, massage, vaporization, skin care, and as a disinfectant.

patchouli

Fragrance—a traditional Indian medicine with a sweet, sensual, earthy, and musky fragrance.

Properties—soothing and uplifting. It is good to use on mature and dry skin.

Beneficial for—quelling apprehension and improving clarity. It is an acknowledged aphrodisiac.

Safety—not suitable for children.

Usage—for bathing, massage, vaporization, and skin care.

peppermint

Fragrance—fresh and cooling.

Properties—refreshing for fatigue as it cools and revives an overheated body. It is also good for clearing headaches.

right: **Pine.**

below left: **Peppermint.**

below right: **Rosemary.**

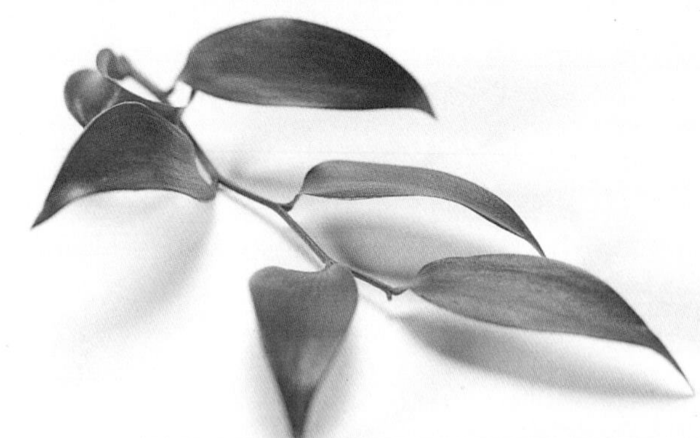

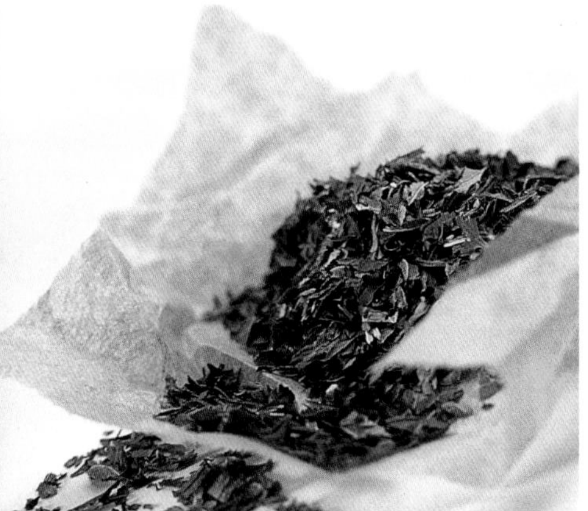

Beneficial for—soothing aches, pains, and stomach upsets, and it is a mental stimulant, so it is revitalizing. It is an ideal substitute for aspirin.

Safety—do not use on sensitive skin, on children, during pregnancy, or when undergoing homeopathic treatment.

Usage—massage, vaporization, foot baths, and as an insect repellent.

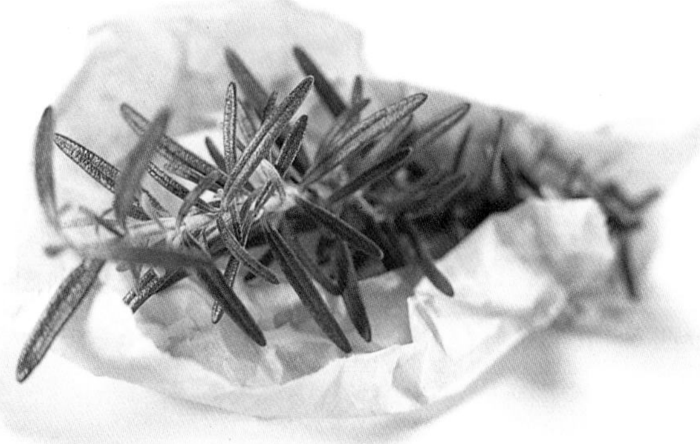

pine

Fragrance—clear and fresh.

Properties—it is a powerful antiseptic, so it is good to use as an inhalant.

Beneficial for—easing bronchitis and respiratory problems.

Safety—do not use during pregnancy.

Usage—for bathing, massage, vaporization, and as a disinfectant.

rose

Fragrance—considered to be the queen of the flower oils, it is expensive and precious. It has an exquisite, sensual, and feminine scent.

Properties—a very feminine oil that is extremely good for regulating period pain and for skin care.

Beneficial for—countering grief, sadness, and regret. It is said that it makes a woman feel good about herself.

Safety—do not use during pregnancy.

Usage—for bathing, massage, vaporization, and skin care.

rosemary

Fragrance—penetrating and stimulating.

Properties—eases tired muscles and aids suppleness. It can heighten concentration and memory and is mentally re-energizing.

Beneficial for—encouraging assertion, focus, and drive. It is a good tonic for dandruff, a hangover, and for a poor circulation.

Safety—do not use during pregnancy.

Usage—for bathing, massage, vaporization, skin care, and foot baths.

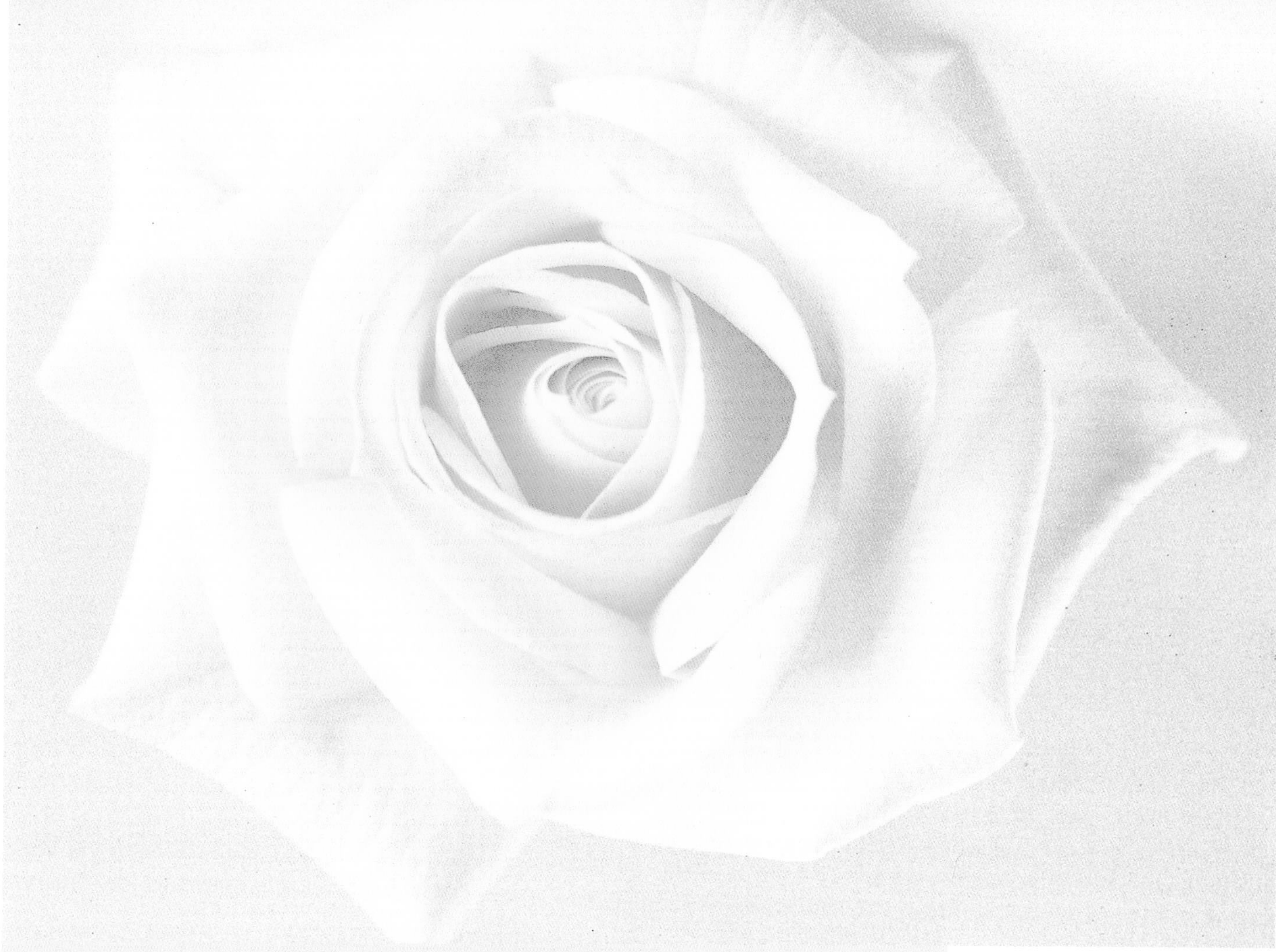

above: **Rose.**

tea tree

Fragrance—strong medicinal smell that is invigorating and antiseptic.

Properties—it is anti-bacterial, anti-fungal, stimulating, and good for the immune system.

Beneficial for—problem skin and for cleansing the skin. Its restorative qualities make it very useful in the sick room.

Safety—Check with your physician before using on sensitive skin.

Usage—for bathing, massage, vaporization, skin care, and as an insect repellent.

ylang-ylang

Fragrance—exotic, sensual, and languid.

Properties—it is both calming and uplifting, and it is known to be a spiritual oil. It is excellent for skin care and also aids peaceful sleep.

Beneficial for—instilling confidence and encouraging expression. It is used as an aphrodisiac in Indonesia, where petals are traditionally scattered over the newlyweds' bed to encourage romance.

Safety—not suitable for children.

Usage—for bathing, massage, vaporization, and skin care.

chapter 4

scent w

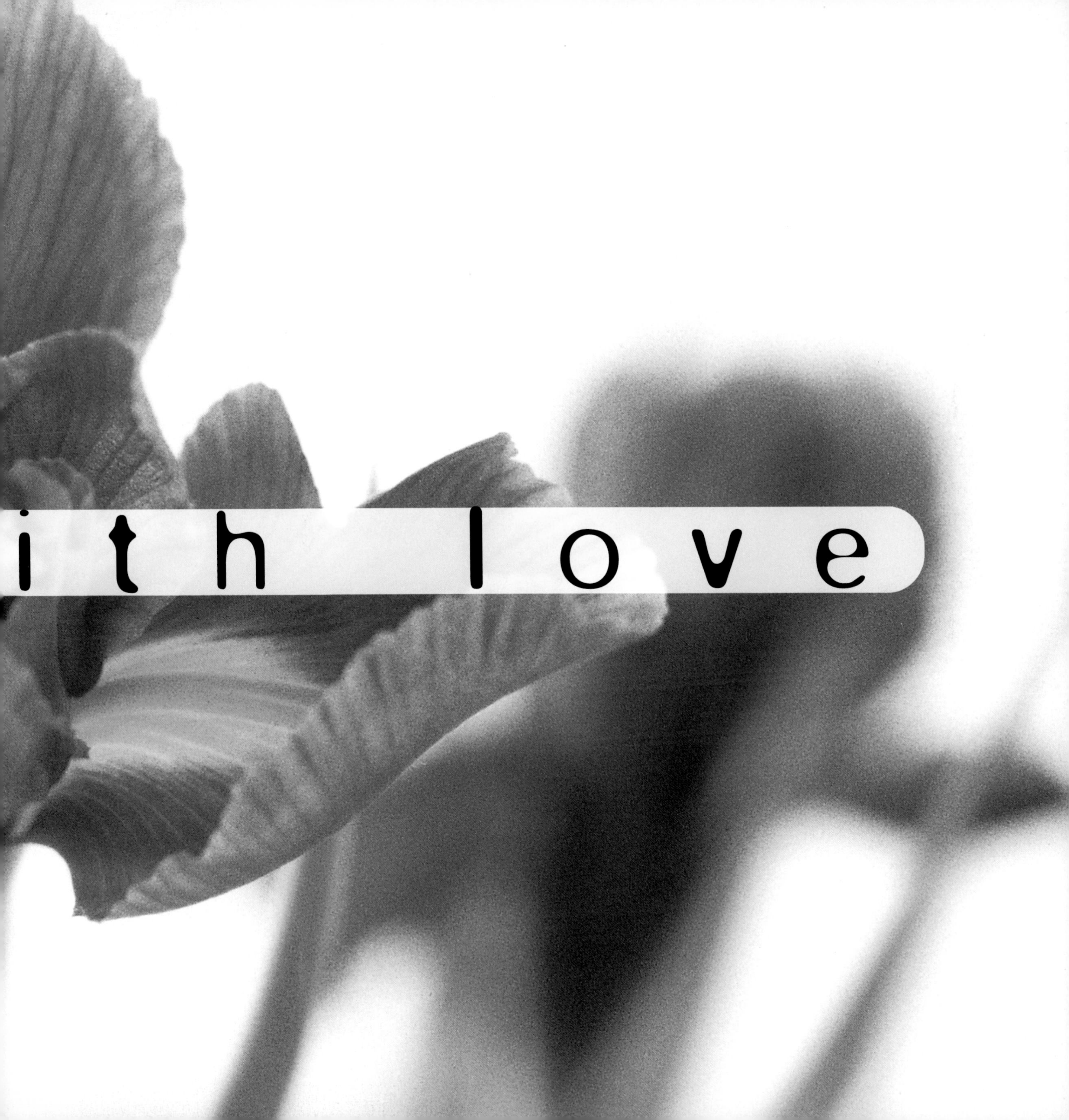
ith love

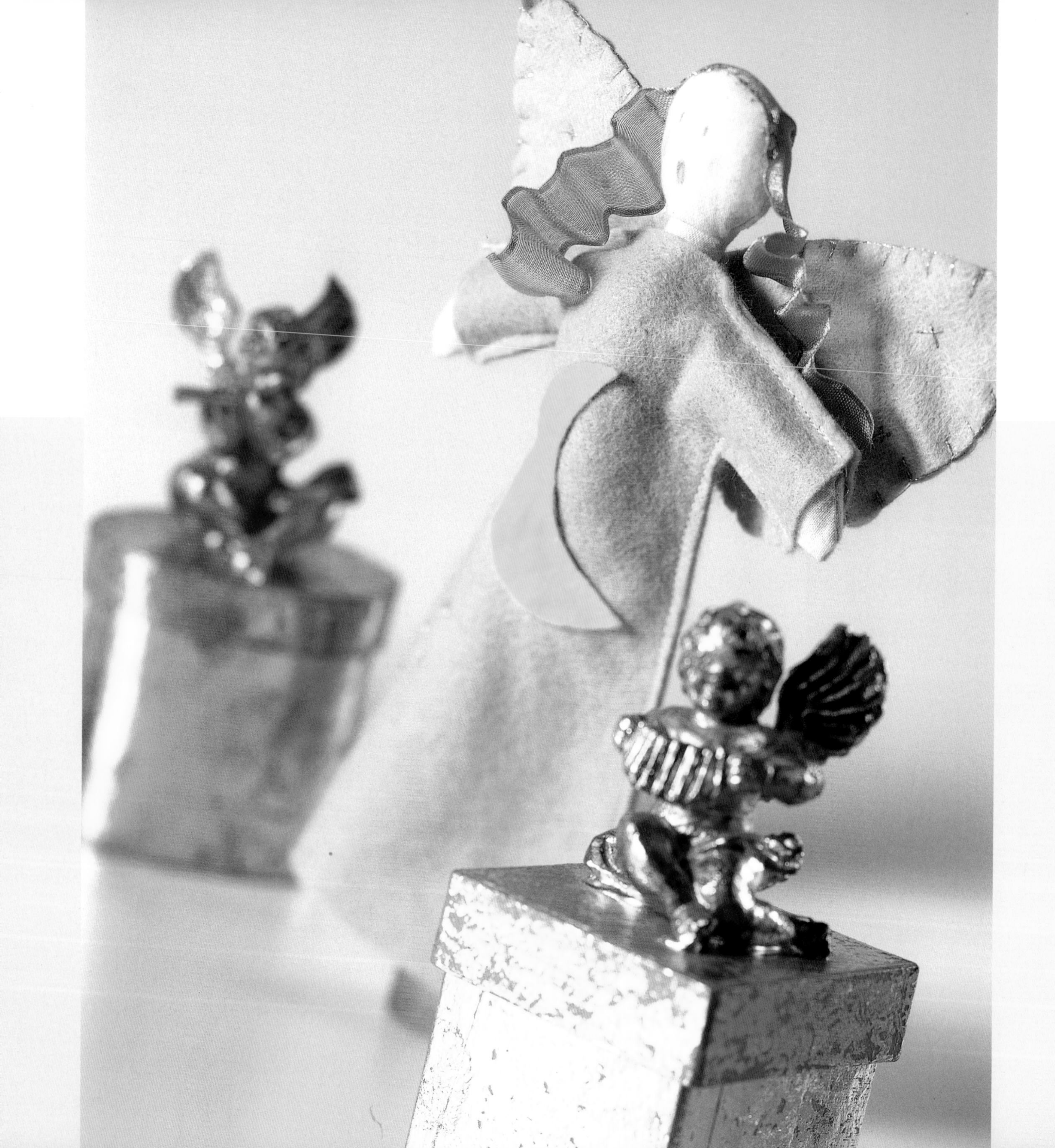

ANGELIC JASMINE AROMA

This calico and felt angel is scented with precious jasmine essential oil. It makes a delightful Christmas tree ornament—the jasmine complementing the pine fragrance of the tree. It would make a lovely doll for a child, or can be used to scent a closet.

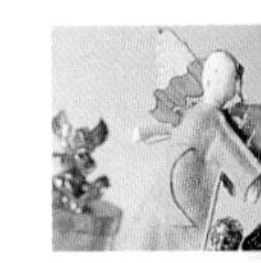

you will need

scissors
unbleached calico
gray, blue, and yellow felt
sewing machine
sewing needle
white and blue sewing thread
polyester batting (wadding)
bowl
orris root powder
jasmine essential oil
fabric glue
gold embroidery thread
pale pink- and blue-colored pencils
gold wired ribbon

one

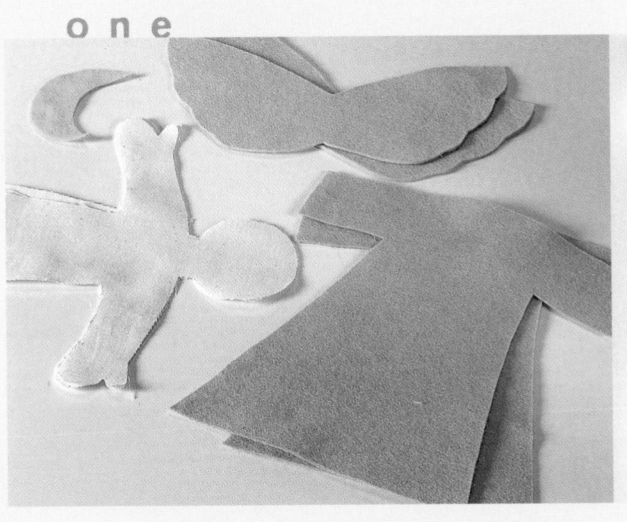

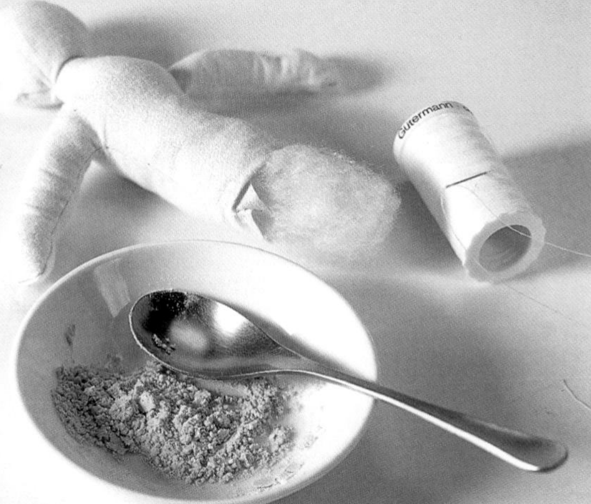

two

step 1 Using the templates on pages 138 and 139, cut out two angels in muslin, two wings in gray felt, and two dresses in blue felt. Cut a small crescent moon in yellow felt for the motif on the angel's dress.

step 2 In a bowl blend 2 rounded teaspoons of orris root powder with 4 to 5 drops of jasmine essential oil, then put aside. Machine or hand-sew together the two pieces of the angel's body with the white thread, leaving only the bottom edge open. Turn right side out and stuff with batting, ensuring that the hands, arms, and head are filled. Sprinkle the exposed batting with the orris root and jasmine mixture. Hand-stitch the opening closed.

three

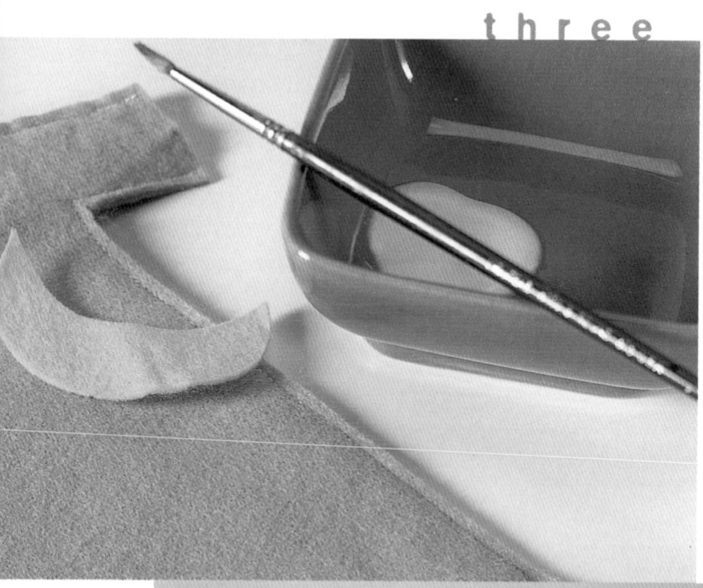

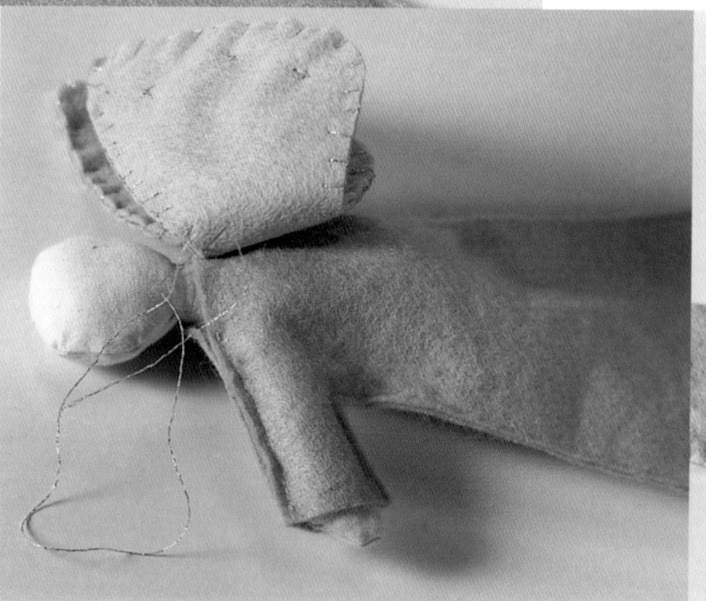

four

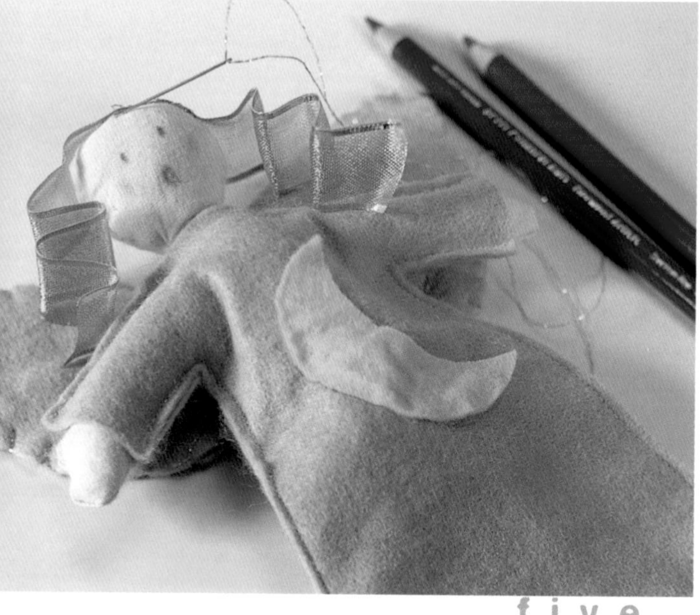

five

step 3 Using a small running stitch, machine stitch the two pieces of the dress together with the blue thread. Leave openings at the neck, sleeve holes, and bottom edge. Pull the dress over the body to glue the moon onto the bodice.

step 4 Sew the two wing pieces together using gold embroidery thread and a blanket stitch. Add details to the wings with cross-stitch. Using the gold thread, sew the wings onto the back of the angel, as shown.

step 5 Draw a simple face onto the angel using pale pink and blue colored pencils. Take a length of wired gold ribbon and crimp it to make the angel's hair. Sew it into place along the crown of the head.

GORGEOUS GIFT-WRAPPING

Here are four stunning ways to wrap and decorate your gifts to make them highly personalized. In each, a scent is used that will imbue any gift-giving occasion with special meaning.

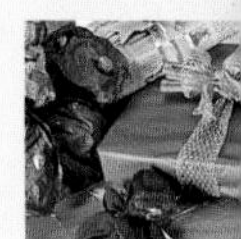

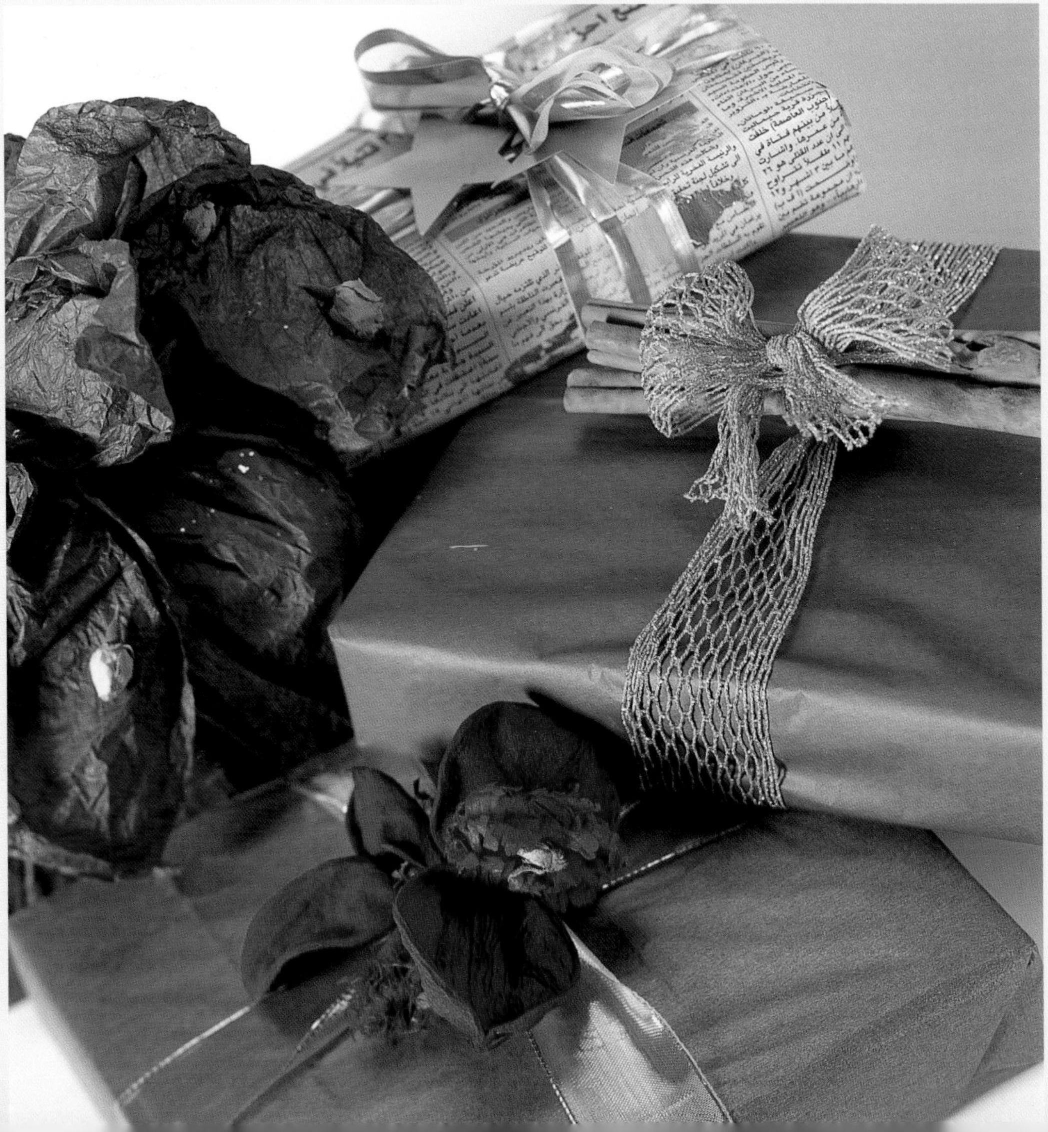

you will need

scissors

clear tape

selection of green tissue paper

cinnamon sticks

gold mesh ribbon

dried rosebuds

white craft glue

glitter

iridescent ribbon

gold embroidery thread and needle

dried potpourri rose petals

newspaper

gold leaf

silver ribbon

silver card

geranium essential oil

hole punch

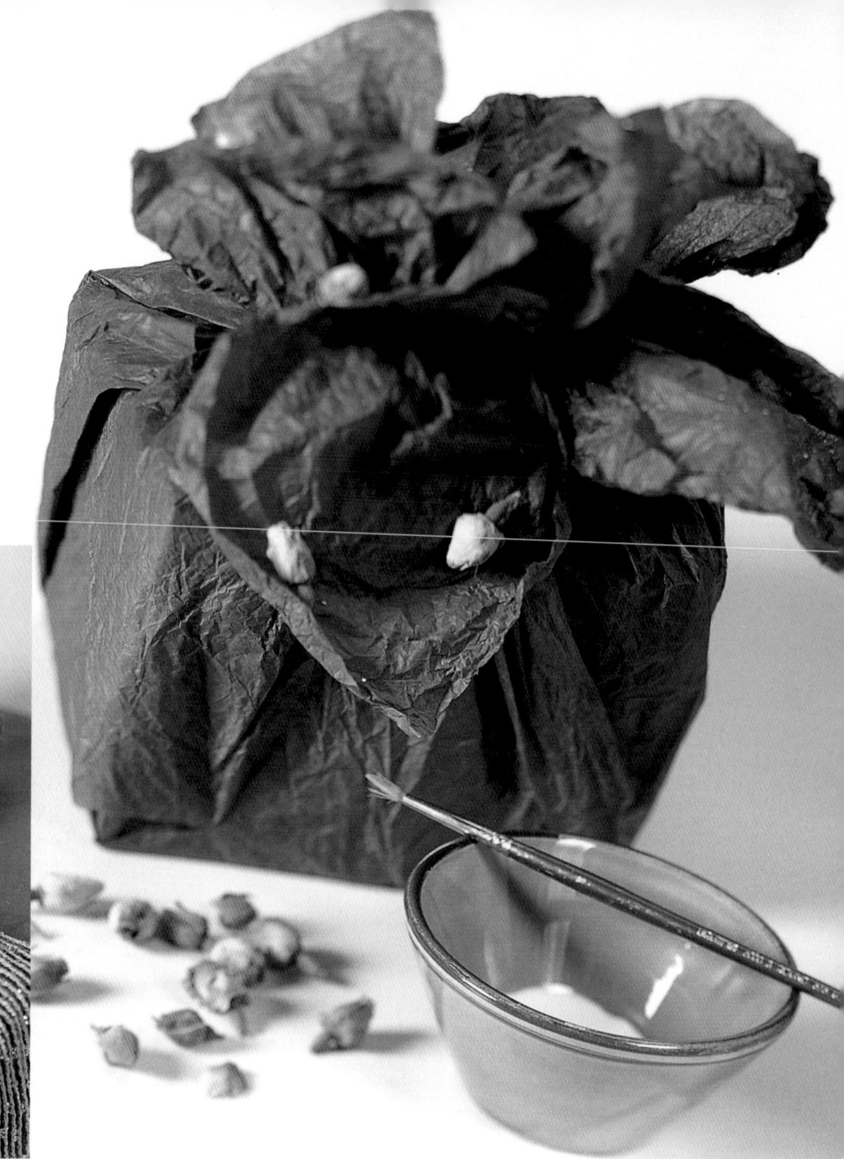

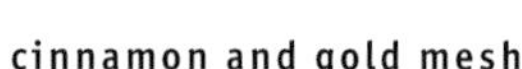

cinnamon and gold mesh

Wrap the gift with dark green tissue paper. Tie a bundle of cinnamon sticks together with gold mesh ribbon, and finish with an elaborate bow. Attach the cinnamon sticks to the front of the gift with more gold mesh ribbon.

exotic bloom

Lay one square of dark green tissue paper onto a flat surface. Lay a square of lighter green tissue paper on top and turn it through 45 degrees (for rectangular pieces of tissue, turn the top sheet through 90 degrees). Place the gift in the center. Pull the corners of both pieces of tissue toward the top center of the gift. Carefully bind them together at the bottom with clear tape. Tease out each corner to create a flamboyant, organic shape. Decorate with dried rosebuds attached on with glue. Finish with a light sprinkling of glitter.

potpourri posies

Wrap the gift in shiny green tissue paper and iridescent ribbon, as shown. Carefully sew together dried potpourri rose petals with gold embroidery thread. Use the thread to attach the petal posies to the ribbon.

newspaper and gold leaf

Cover the gift with newspaper—one in a foreign language always looks interesting—or other printed paper. Apply glue to some areas and, while still wet, press on small pieces of gold leaf. When dry, tie the gift with silver ribbon. To make a gift tag, cut a star from silver card and apply a few drops of geranium essential oil to the back. Punch a hole into the star and attach to the gift with a length of silver ribbon. Curl the ribbon by running it firmly across one blade of some scissors.

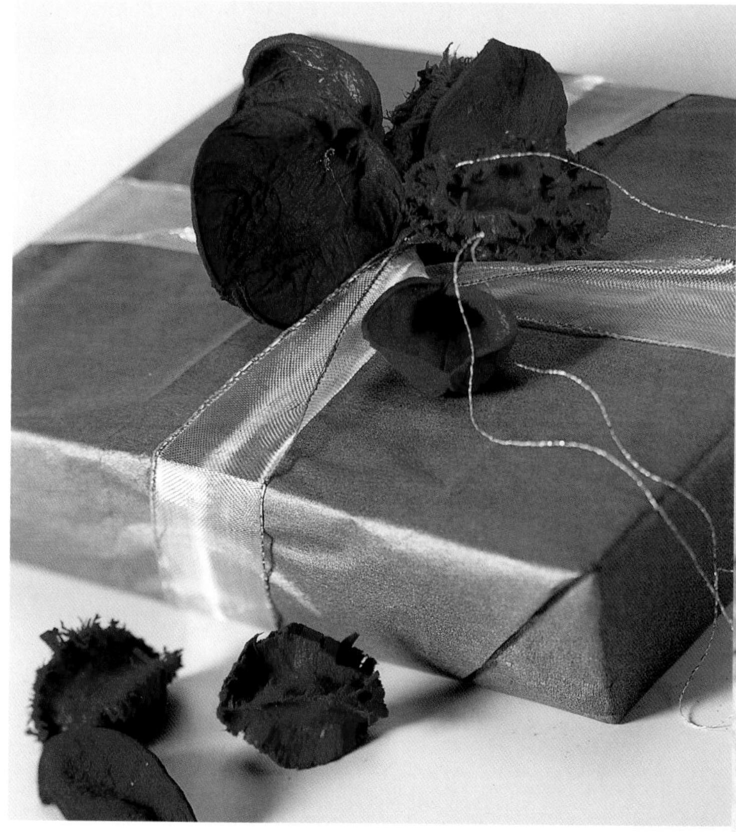

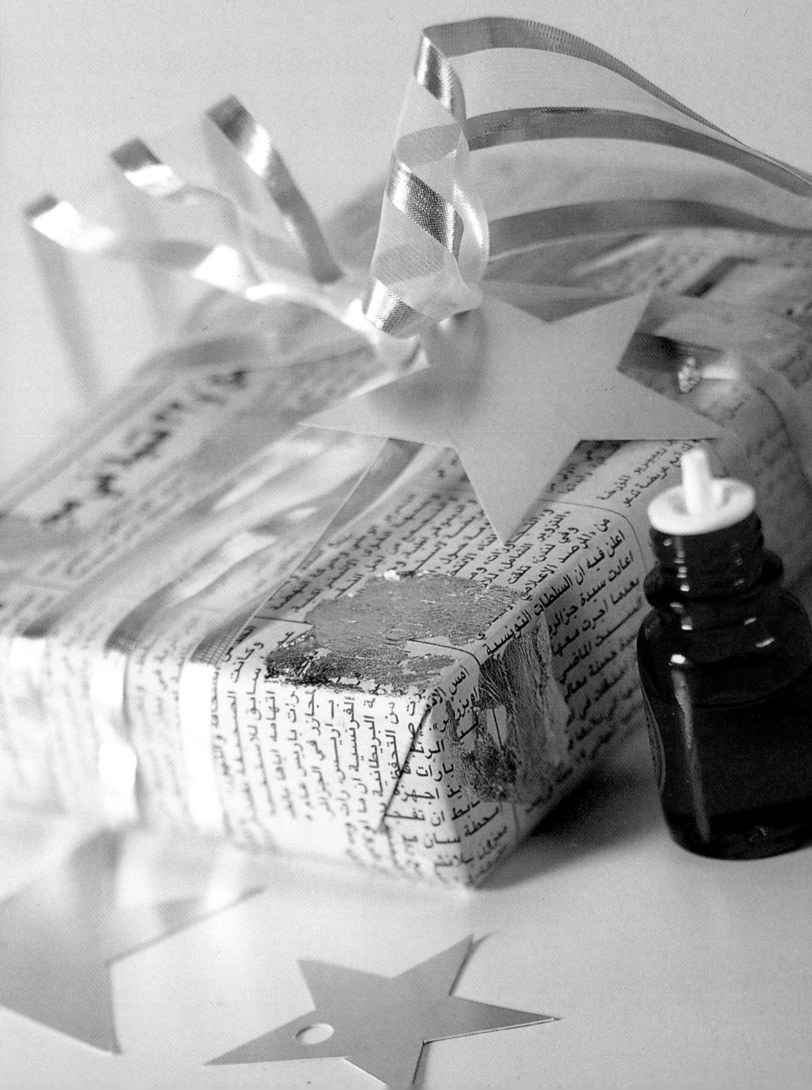

PEPPERMINT GIFT TAGS

Use beautiful Japanese ichimatsu paper, folded and glued to hold scented cards and hologram sequins, to make a paper sachet that slips inside an envelope to imbue a letter or card with a memorable fragrance.

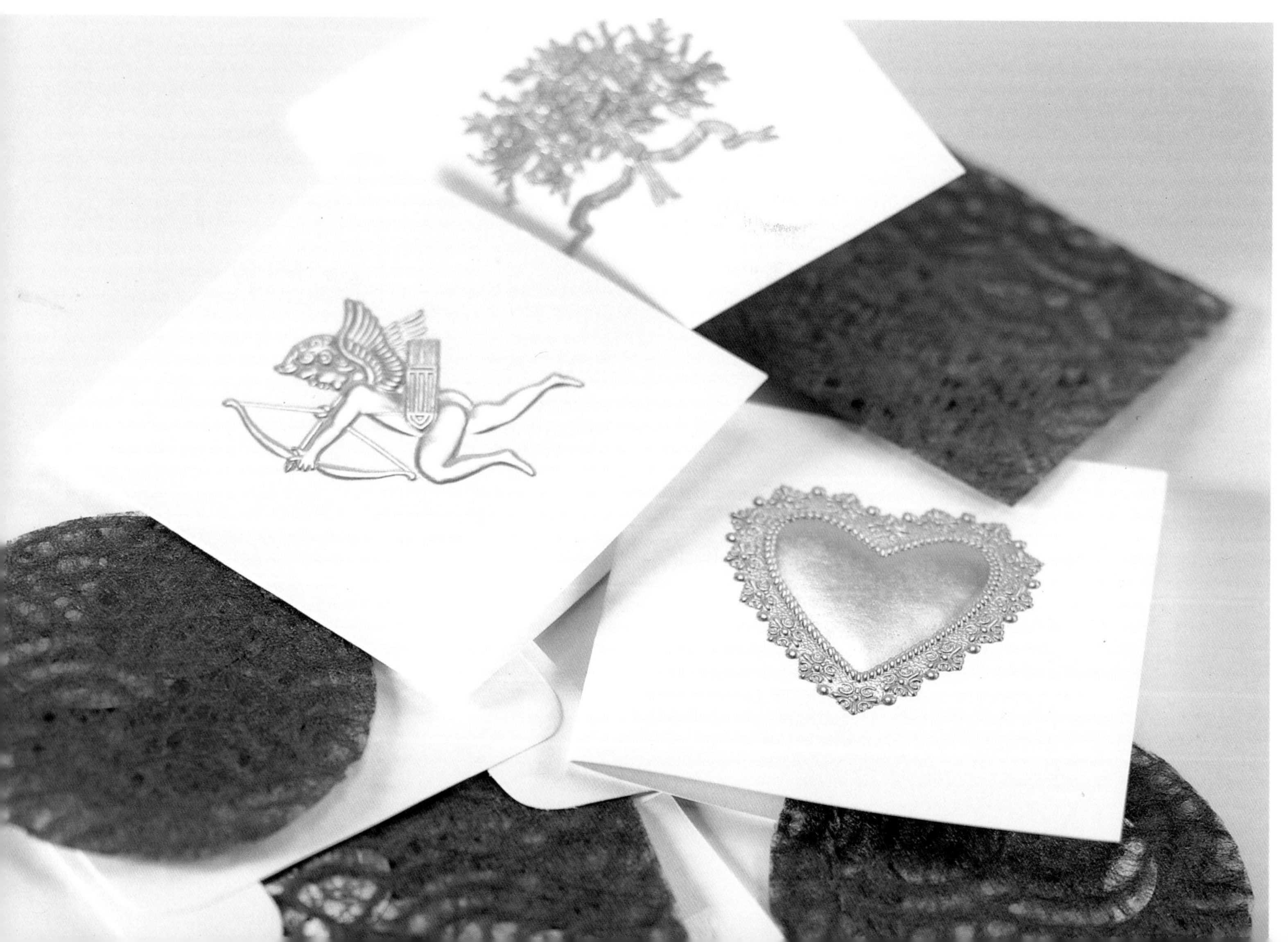

step 1 Cut the Japanese paper into a 6-inch by 3-inch rectangle. Fold it in half lengthways. Join two edges with glue to form an almost-square sachet with an opening. To make a round sachet, trace around the lid of a jar onto the Japanese paper and cut out two circles. Partially join the circles by applying glue to the edge of only one half of the circles, leaving a wide opening.

step 2 Using a large coin as a template, draw around it onto the back of the copper-colored card. You will need one or two circles of card for each sachet. Cut out the circles with sharp scissors. Apply one drop of peppermint oil onto the back of each circle. The oil will leave a greasy mark, so take care not to get it on the front of the card. To conceal this mark, stick two circles together, wrong sides facing, after applying the oil.

step 3 Place one or two scented circles and some large, colorful round sequins into each sachet. Seal openings with glue. Allow to dry before enclosing a sachet inside an envelope.

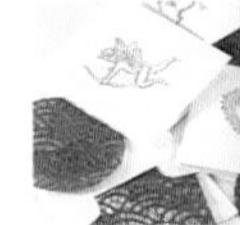

you will need

scissors

Japanese ichimatsu paper or any hand-made porous paper

white glue

large coin

copper-colored card

peppermint essential oil

large round hologram

sequins in various colors

one

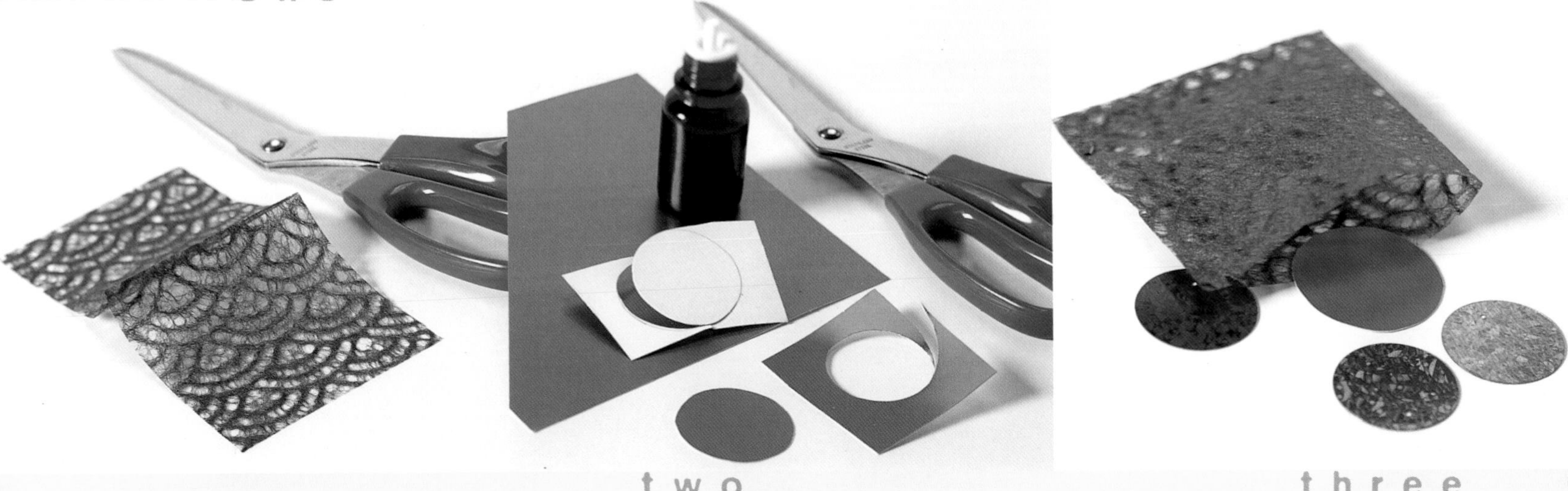

two

three

SCENTED PAPER ROLL

Rather than scenting sheets of note paper individually, make a padded roll that can be used time and time again. Simply wrap a few sheets of note paper around the roll, which has been filled with wadding, preservatives, and essential oil, and allow the paper to absorb the scent.

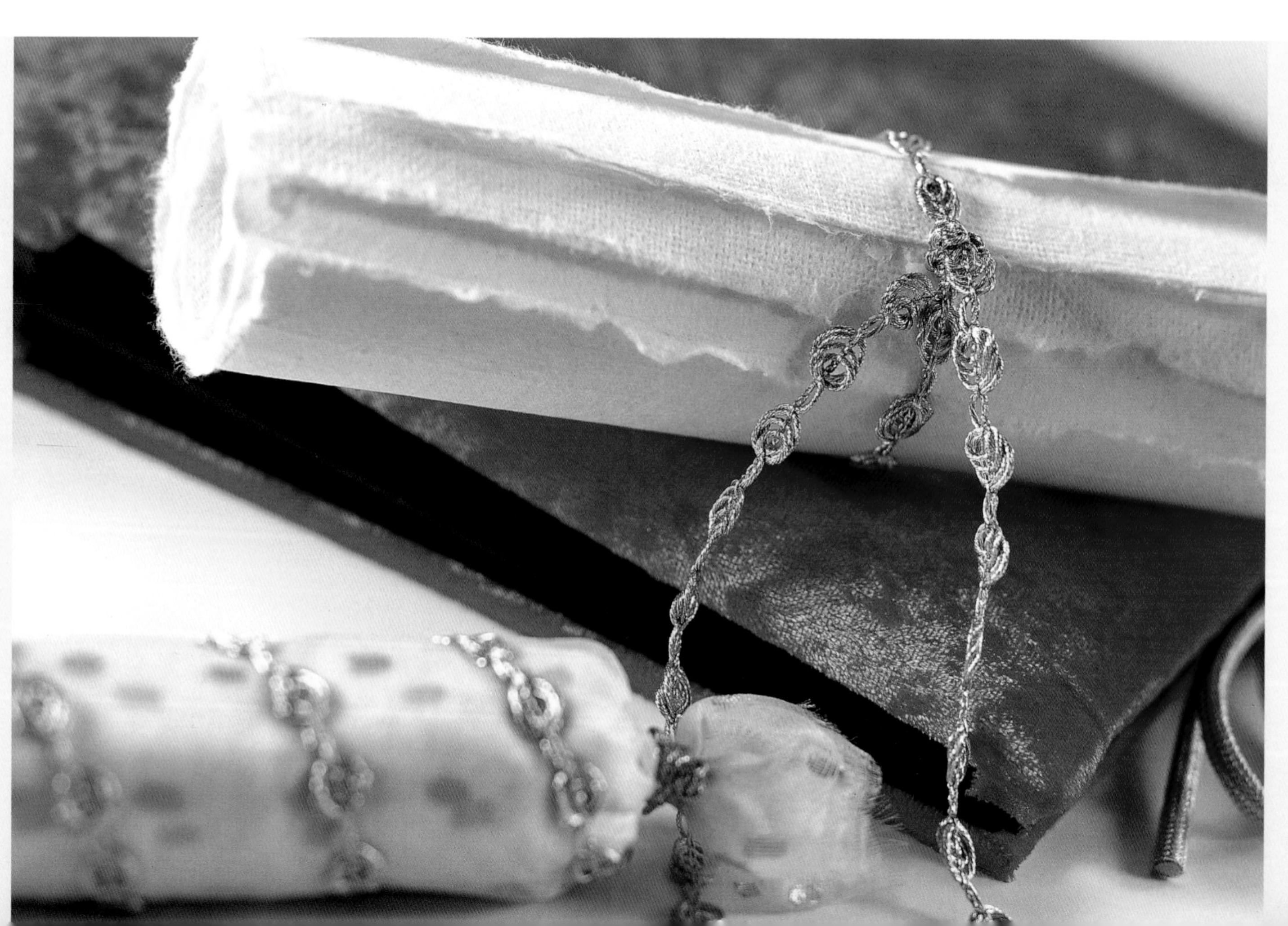

step 1 In a very small bowl, mix four teaspoons of orris root powder with ten drops of gum benzoin. Add six drops each of cedarwood and sandalwood essential oils and mix thoroughly. This mixture is sufficient for one scented roll.

step 2 Place the square of cotton fabric onto a flat surface. Position the rectangle of wadding onto one half of the square. Sprinkle the scented mixture evenly onto the wadding.

step 3 Roll the cotton fabric and the wadding to form a sausage shape, and secure the overlapping edge with pins. Fold over the ends and fix them in place with glue. Remove the pins and seal the overlapping edge with glue.

step 4 Wrap the organza around the scented roll, tying the ends with gold embroidery thread to resemble a bon-bon or Christmas favor. Finish by winding a long length of decorative gold braid around the roll. Secure the braid by knotting it around the ends, as shown. Trim to neaten.

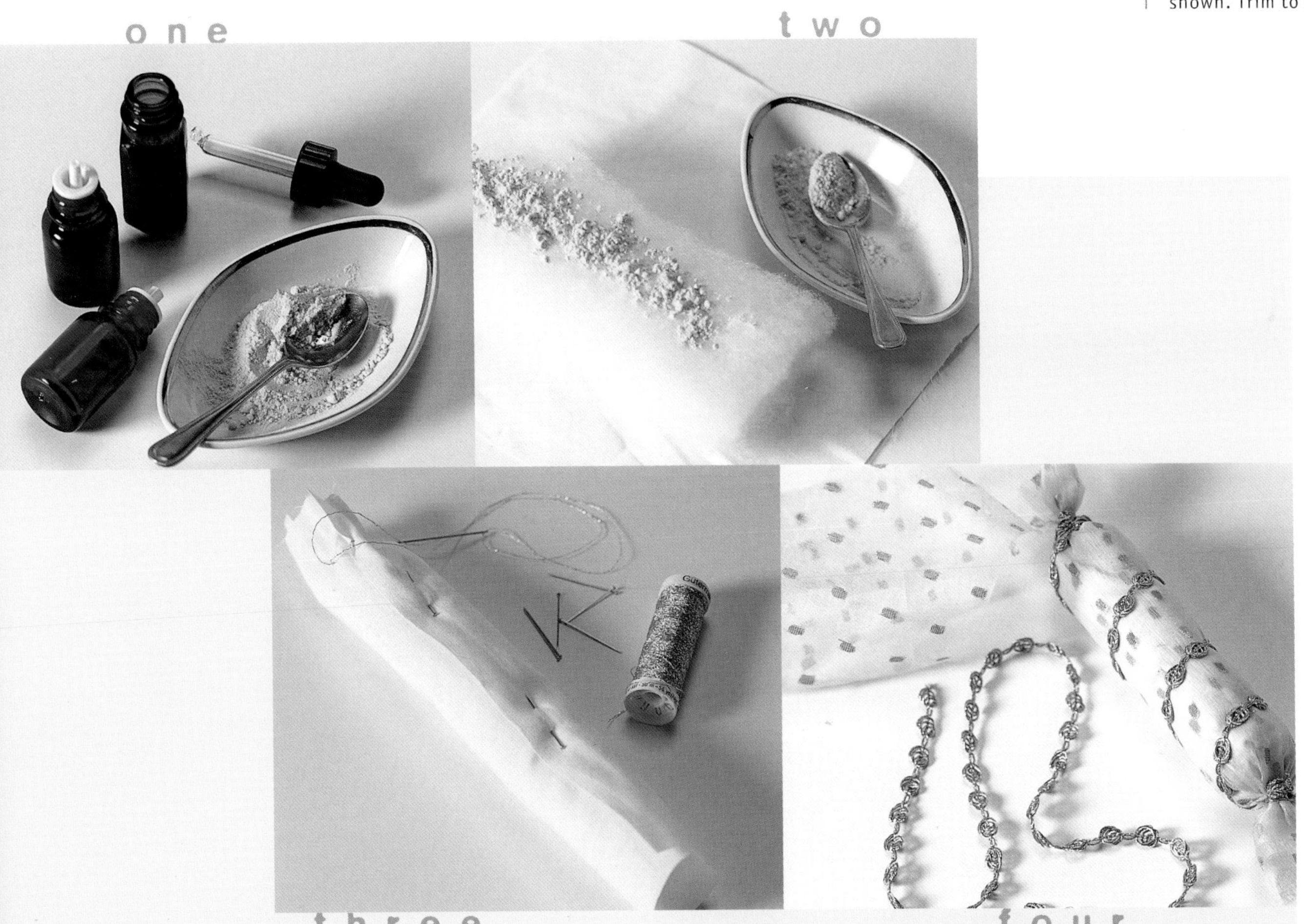

you will need

very small bowl

small mixing spoon

orris root powder

gum benzoin tincture

cedarwood and sandalwood essential oils

7-inch square of cotton fabric

5½ inch by 2½ inch rectangle of wadding

dress-making pins

fabric glue

8-inch square of white embroidered organza

gold embroidery thread

decorative gold braid

EMBOSSED PAPER

Emboss beautiful hand-made note paper that you can then scent on the fragrant paper roll. Embossing requires dampening the paper and applying pressure to it and the wire motifs beneath, to create textured and patterned note paper that is little short of being a work of art.

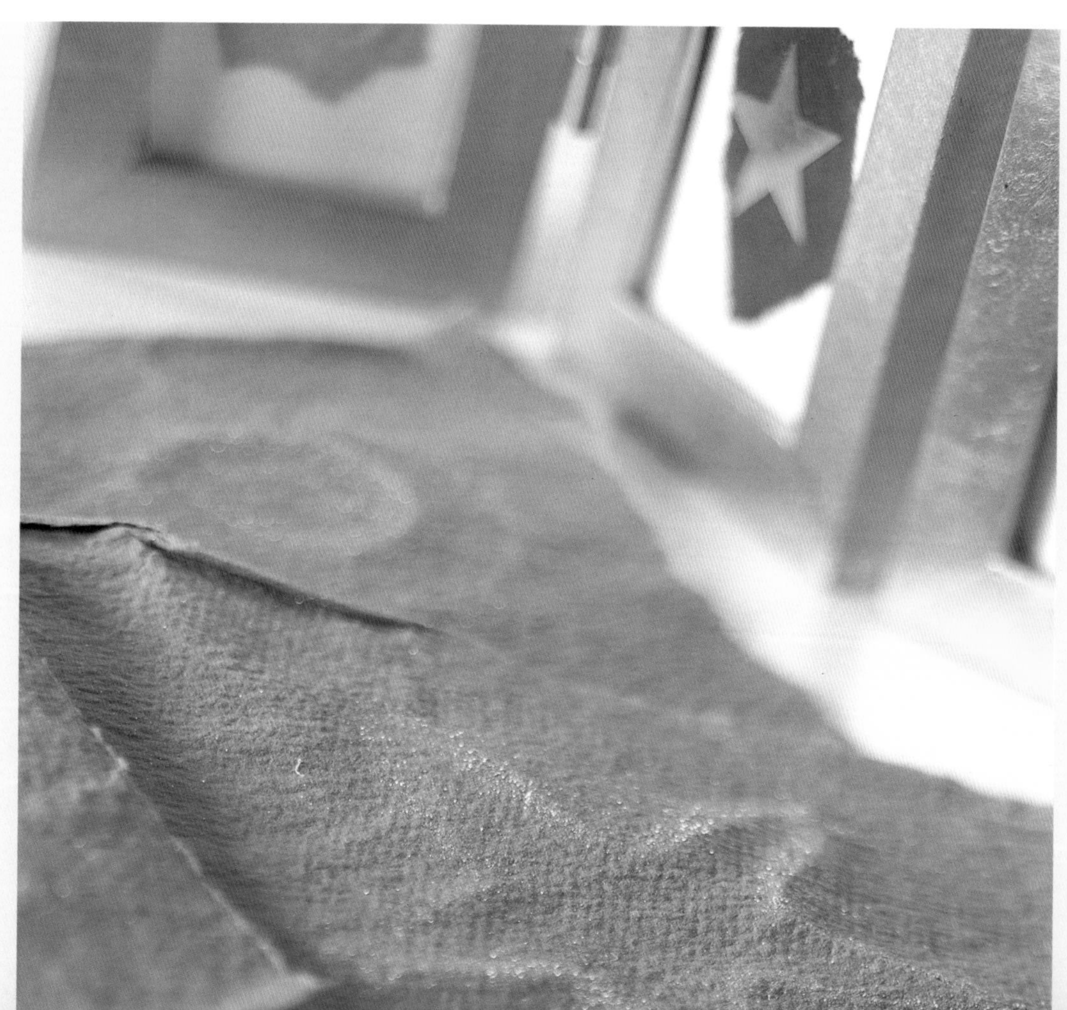

one

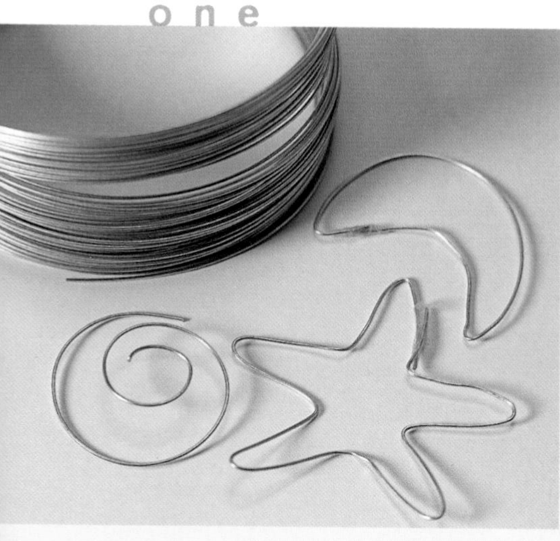

two

three

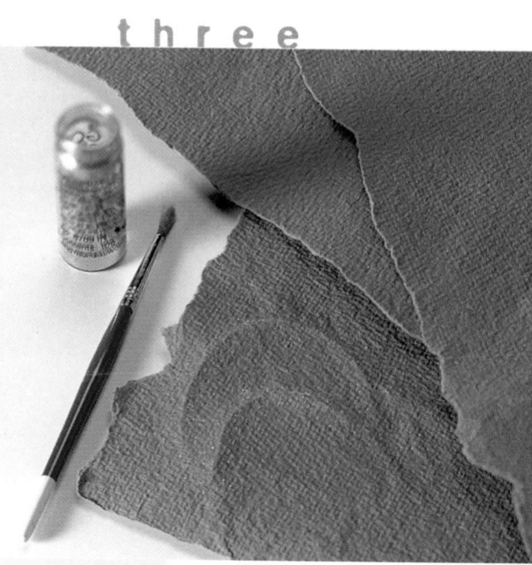

step 1 Cut lengths of wire and bend them (the pliers will help you to make sharp corners) to form a spiral, star, and crescent moon, or motifs of your choice. The templates on page 139 will help you to achieve the right shape. Cut off any excess wire. Fix the free ends of the shaped wire together with tape.

step 2 Using the water spray, dampen the top right-hand corner of the hand-made paper with water. Lay the paper on a flat surface and place the wire shapes directly under the dampened area. Carefully place, so as not to move the paper or the wire, an old woolen blanket on top of the paper. Onto this, place a pile of books. Leave overnight.

step 3 Remove the books and blanket to reveal that the wire shapes have made impressions into the paper. Remove the shapes and lightly brush the embossed (raised) areas with gold powder.

To scent the paper, roll it around the Scented Paper Roll (see page 62) and secure it with ribbon or braid. Allow 2 to 3 hours for the fragrance to permeate the paper.

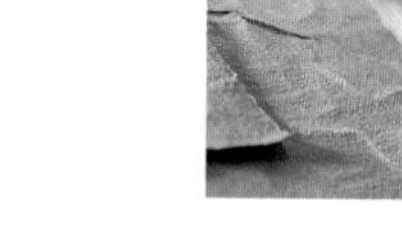

you will need

florists' wire

wire cutters

small pliers

tape

hand-made rag paper

water spray

old woolen blanket or similar

pile of heavy books

gold powder and brush

SCENTED ENVELOPES

The templates at the back of the book, allow you to make highly individual envelopes for your embossed note papers and decorated cards.

You can scent the envelopes to match the enclosure, or give your correspondent a fragrant tour by using complementary scents.

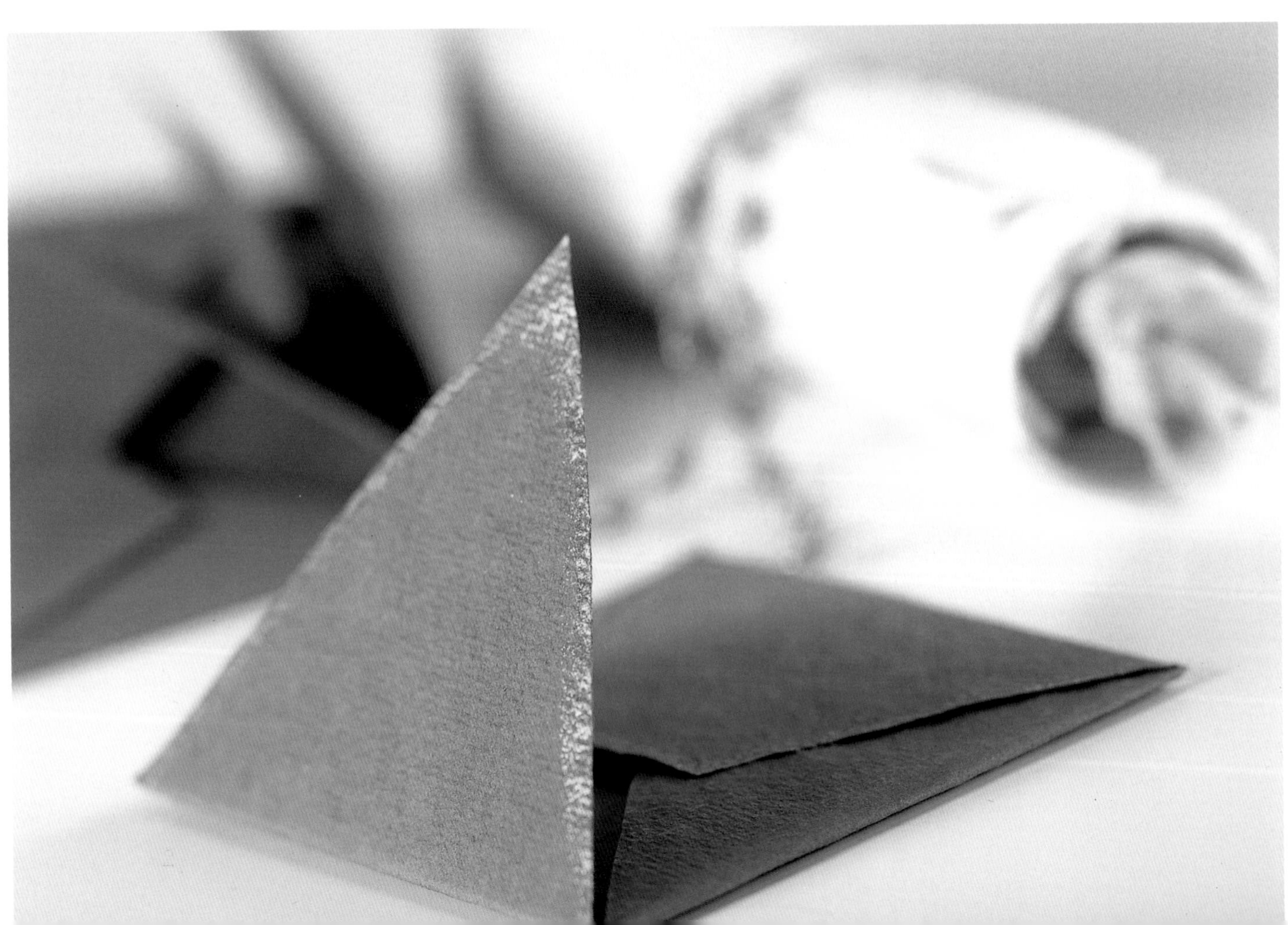

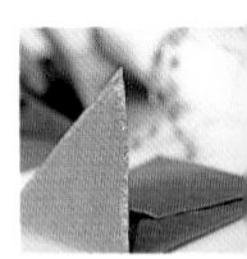

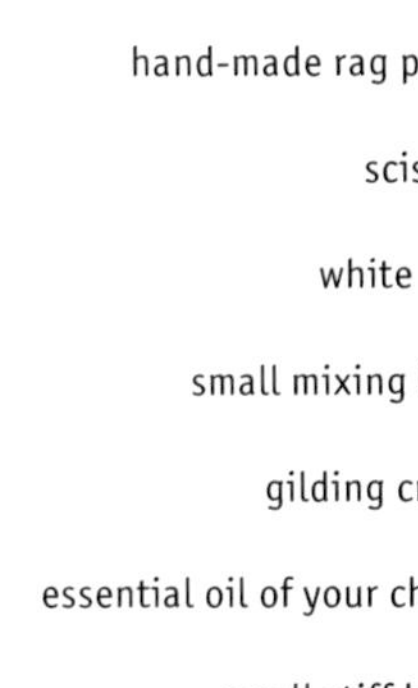

you will need

hand-made rag paper

scissors

white glue

small mixing bowl

gilding cream

essential oil of your choice

small stiff brush
or cotton swab

step 1 Trace and cut out one of the envelope templates on pages 140 and 141. Draw around the template on rag paper. Cut this out and fold, following the dotted lines on the template. Apply glue to the side edges of the bottom flap and press it down firmly onto the two small flaps.

step 2 In a small mixing bowl, thoroughly mix a small amount of gilding cream with a few drops of essential oil so that the oil overpowers the odor of the cream. If you can't smell the essential oil, continue adding more drops of oil.

step 3 To give a burnished look and add a glorious scent, edge the front of the loose flap with the oil and cream mixture. Apply the mixture with a brush or small cotton swab.

one

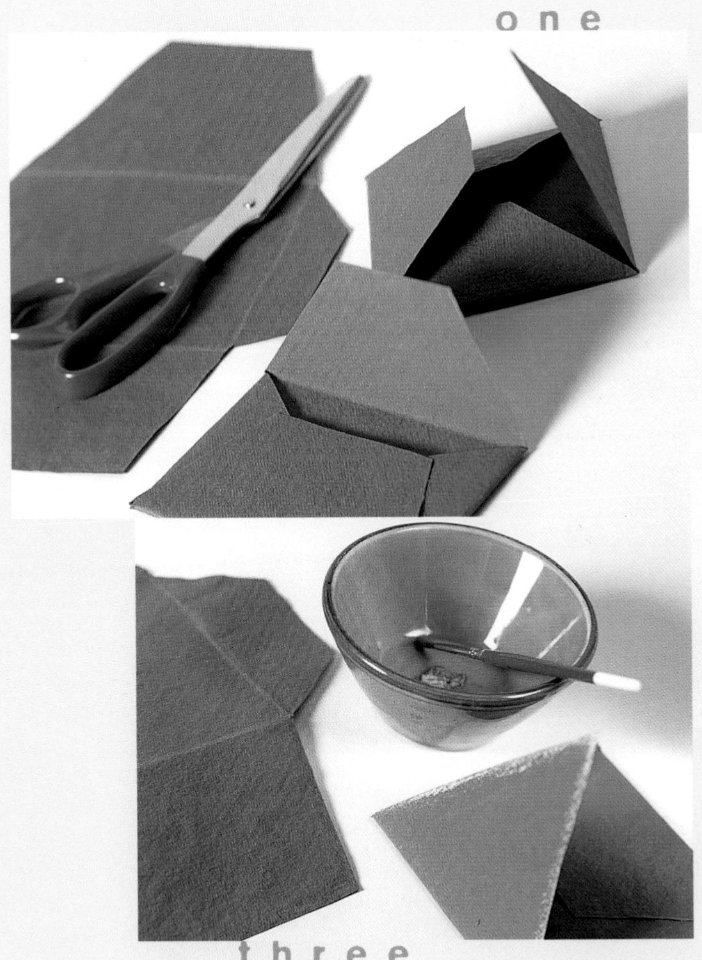

three

two

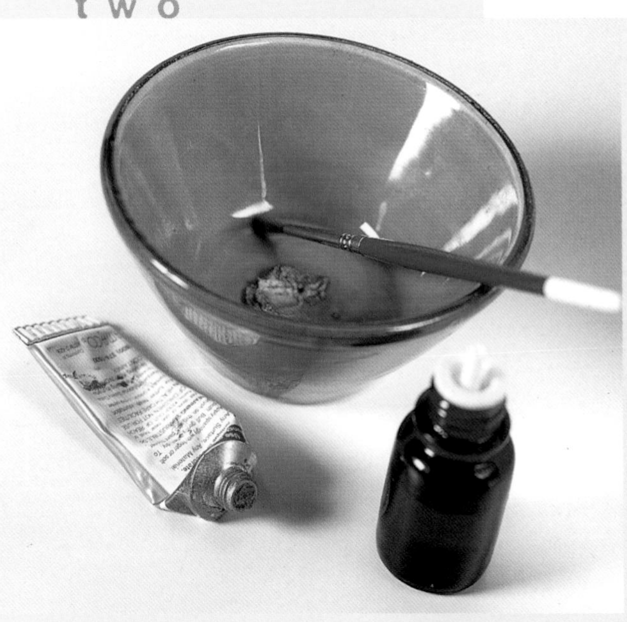

ESSENTIAL OIL CARRIER BOX

Essential oils need to be kept in a cool, dry place, and it is often recommended that they should be boxed and stored away from cosmetics and other perfumes. To this end, here is a decorated and partitioned carrier that will protect your valuable essential oils.

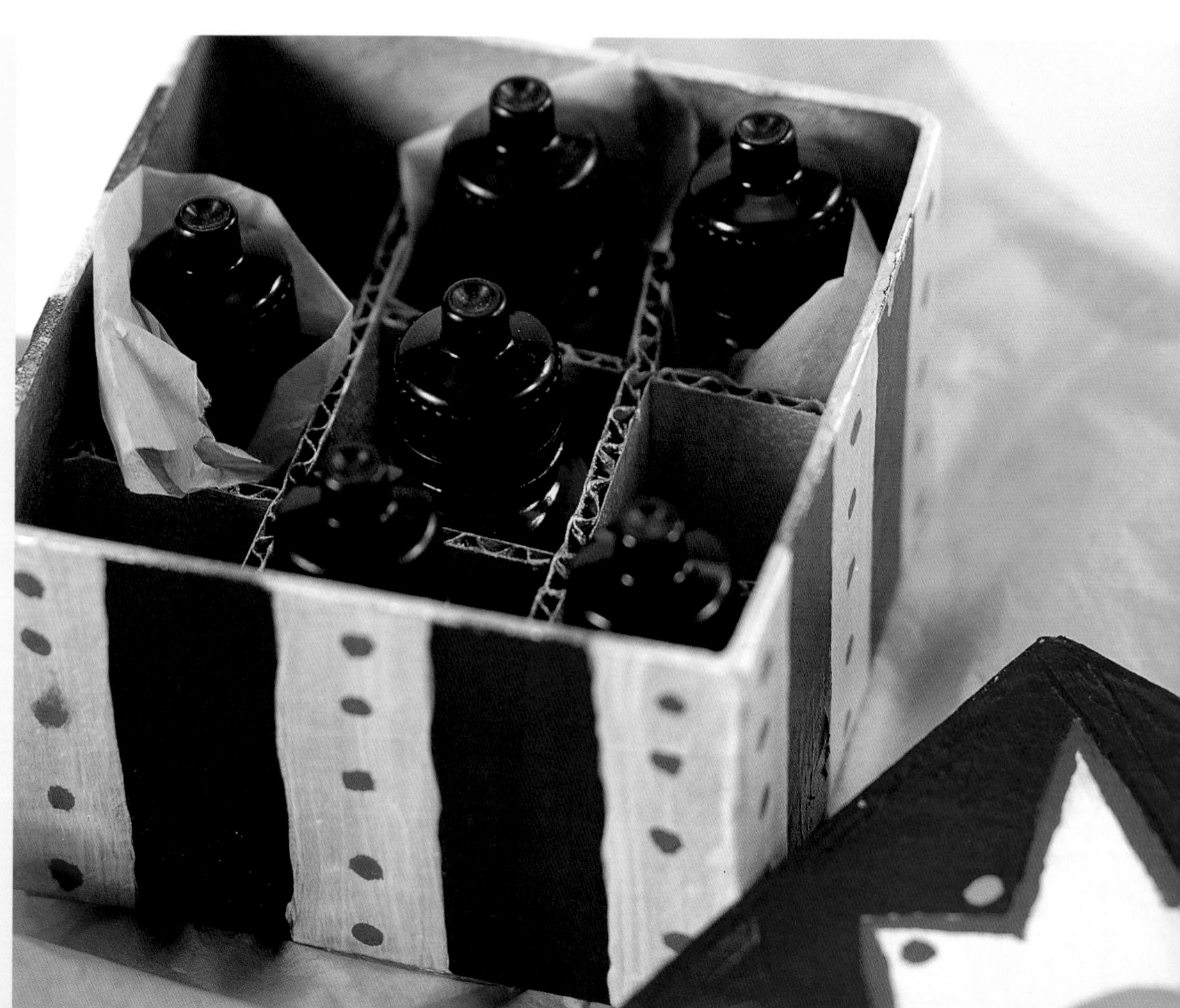

step 1 Draw a simple pattern onto the top and sides of the box using a pencil and faint lines. Paint the design using watercolor or acrylic paints, and let dry.

step 2 Measure and cut four strips of card that are the same length as the box. The width of each strip needs to equal two-thirds of the depth of the box.

step 3 Use a tape measure to divide each strip into thirds. Mark the thirds with lines running to the center of the strip. Cut along the lines. If you are using thick card, as shown, cut two lines side-by-side and remove the narrow pieces of card.

step 4 Slot the strips together to form a grid and place inside the box. This will create nine compartments for essential oil bottles. Spray the grid and the inside of the box silver. Allow to dry.

one

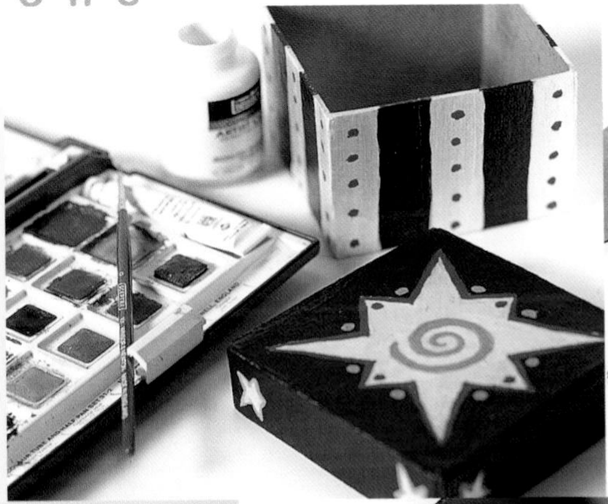

two

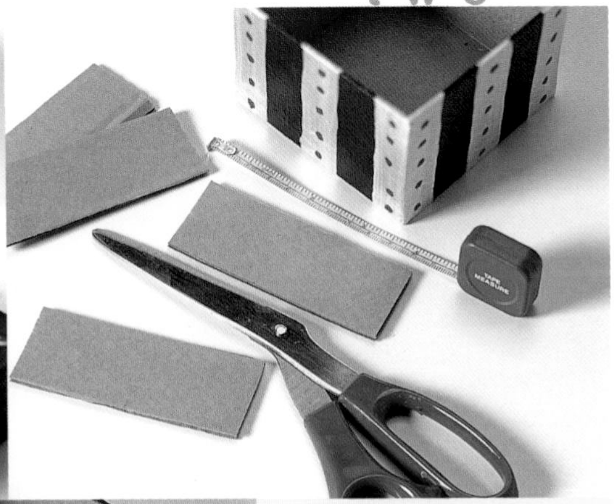

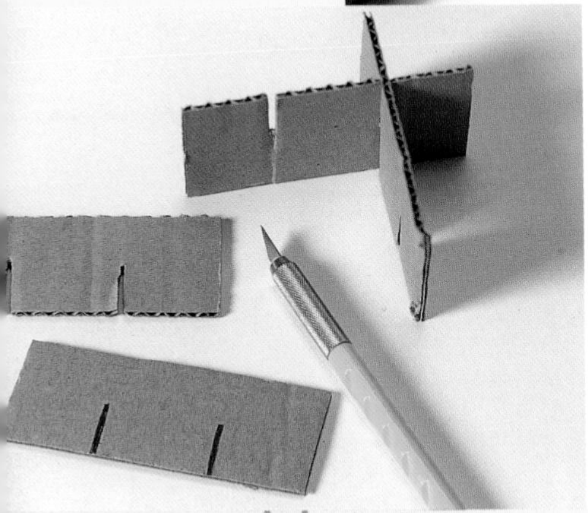

three

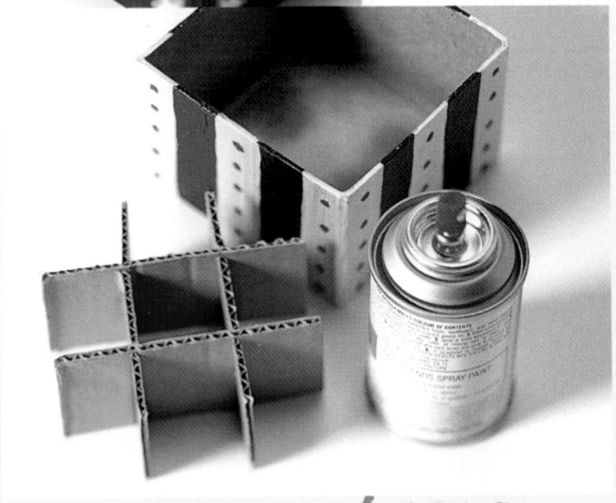

four

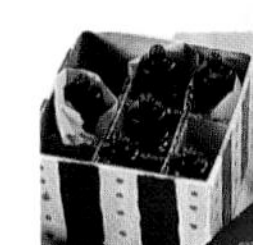

you will need

small square card or papier-mâché box with lid

pencil

watercolor or acrylic paints

fine brushes

thick card

tape measure

scissors or craft knife

silver spray paint

DAISY SACHETS

These very simple sachets, appliquéd in complementary colors, have been filled with dried herbs of eucalyptus, peppermint, and marjoram to give them a fresh and invigorating fragrance.

step 1 Using the pinking shears, cut two identical squares of felt in each of these sizes: $2\frac{1}{2}$-inches square, $3\frac{1}{2}$-inches square, and 5 inches square. Make each pair of squares a different color.

step 2 Cut out three daisies from contrasting felt using the daisy template on page 142. Cut three centers from yellow felt.

step 3 Glue a daisy and a center onto one of the squares in each color. Sew large, simple stitches around the centers using a matching embroidery thread and needle.

step 4 Using the sewing machine set to a small running stitch, sew each pair of squares together, wrong sides facing each other, along three sides. Fill each sachet with a dried herb. Sew the fourth side as before.

one

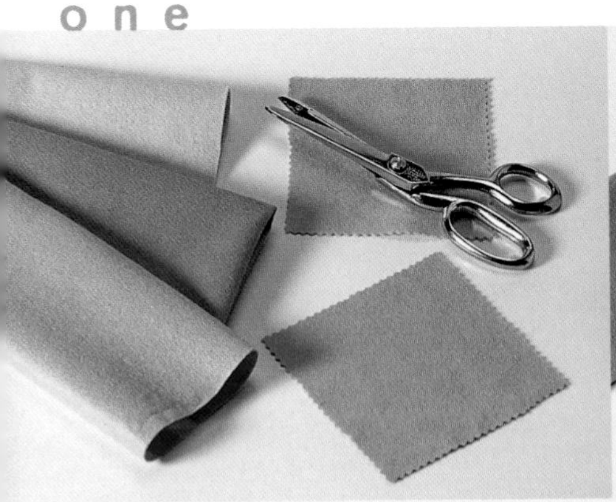

two

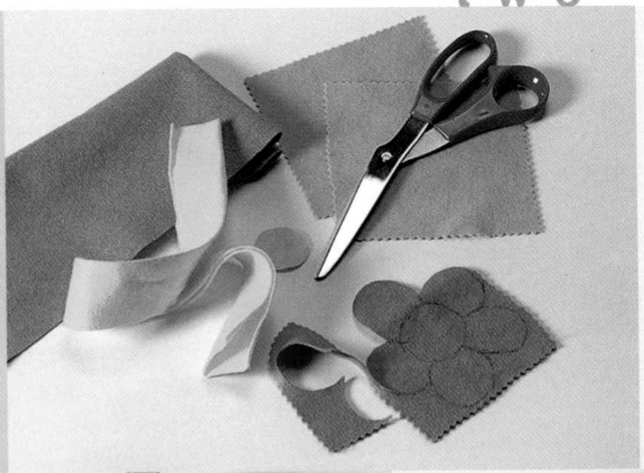

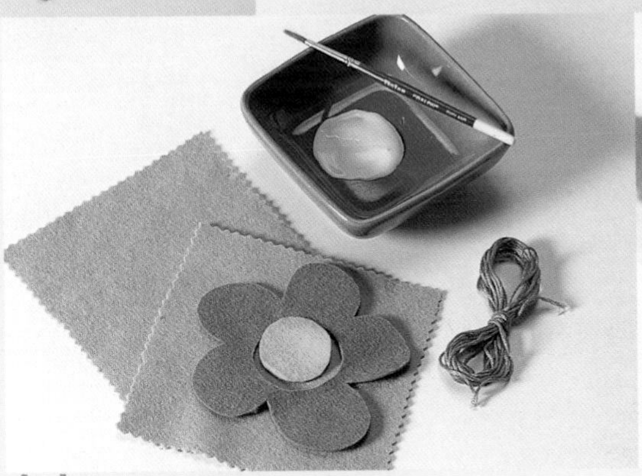

three

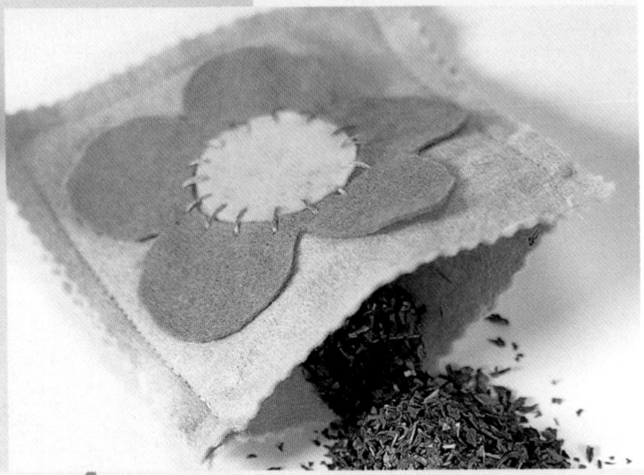

four

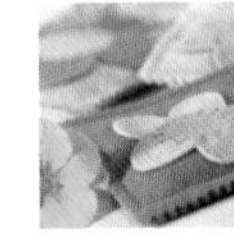

you will need

pinking shears

lilac, gray, blue, and yellow felt

scissors

fabric glue

embroidery thread in lilac, gray, and blue

embroidery needle

sewing machine

sewing thread

dried eucalyptus, peppermint, and marjoram

HEART-SHAPED POTPOURRI BOX

The gold mesh cut-out on the lid of this velvet-covered box reveals the dewberry potpourri inside. It is a perfect place in which to hide treasured keepsakes and Valentine's Day mementos.

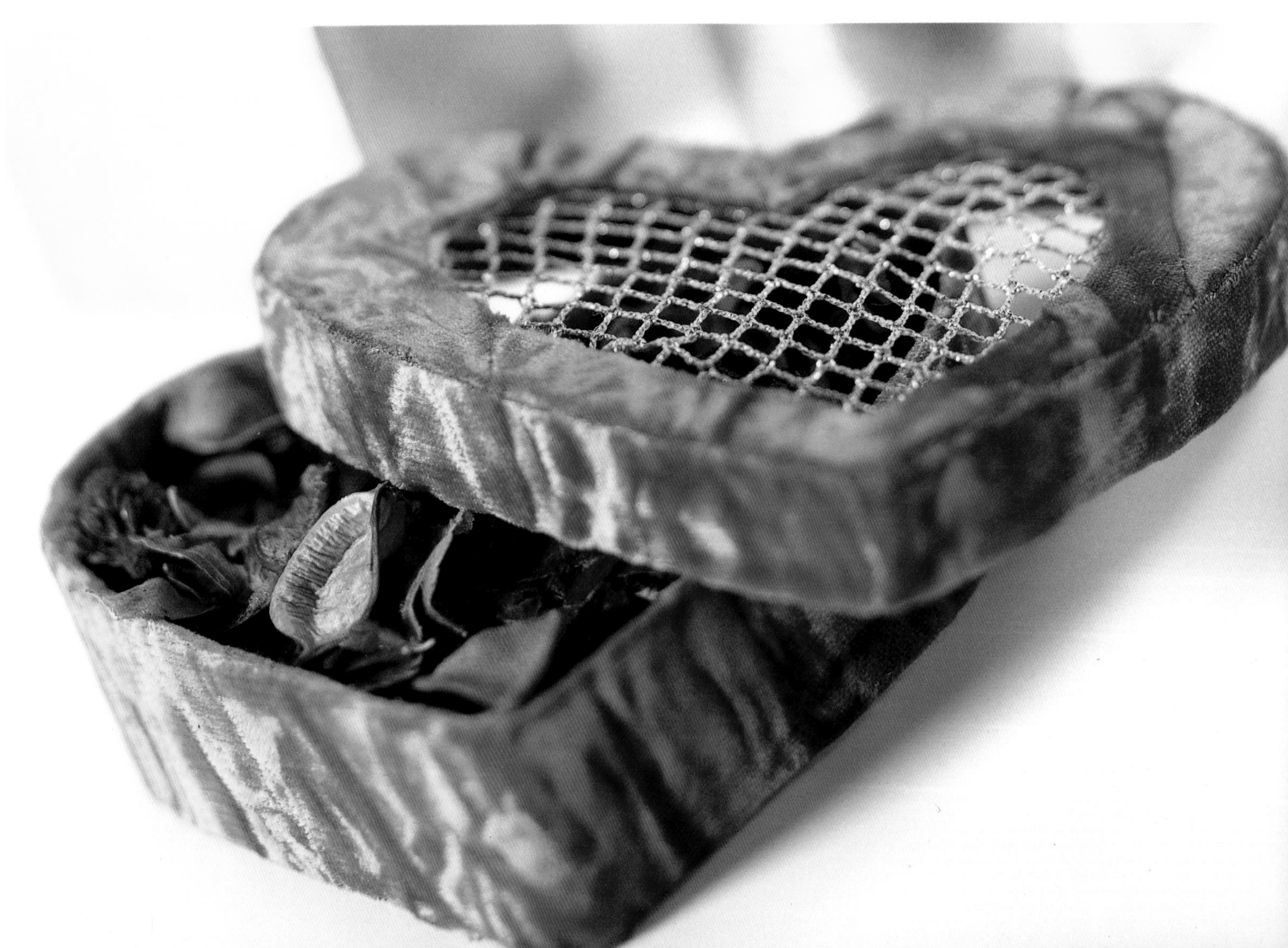

one two three

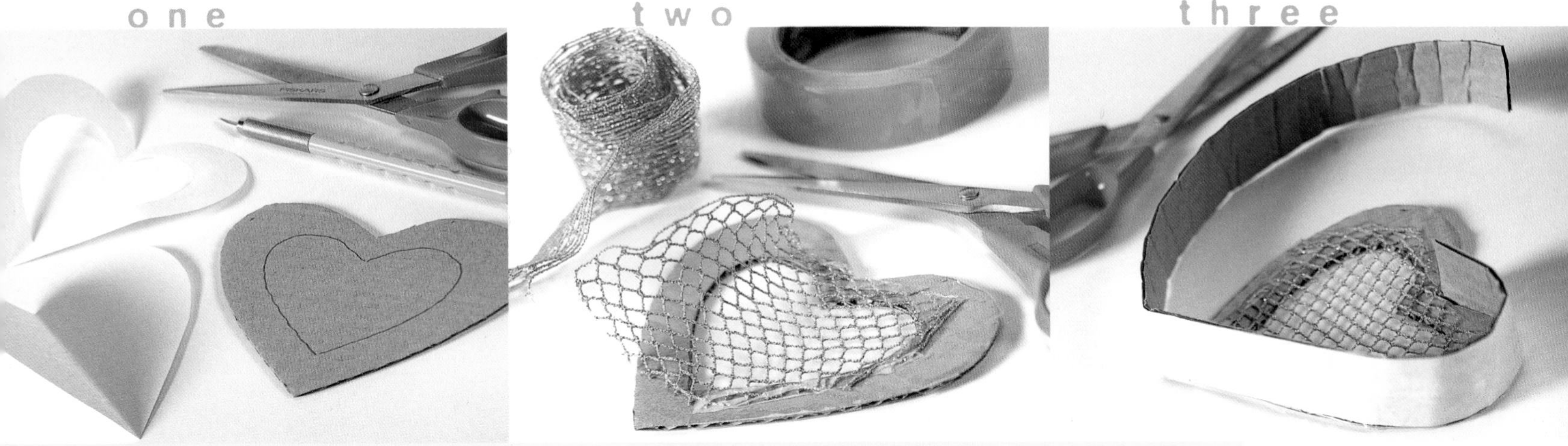

step 1 Trace the three heart templates on page 143 onto paper and cut out and use as templates. The largest heart is for the lid, the medium one for the base of the box, and the smallest one for the cut-out on the lid.

To make the lid, trace around the largest heart onto corrugated cardboard. Position the smallest heart inside this outline and trace around it. Cut out the large heart, then the small one to form the cut-out. Make a tracing of this cut-out so that you can use it later.

Trace around the remaining heart template onto corrugated cardboard and cut it out. This is the base of the box.

step 2 Stretch the gold mesh and place it onto the cut-out. Keeping the mesh taut, secure it firmly in place with tape. Cut off any excess mesh.

step 3 To make the rim of the lid, cut out a strip of corrugated cardboard 18 inches long and ½ inch wide. Position the strip of card around the lid, as shown, and secure it in place with tape applied to the outside of the rim and lid.

To make the side of the base, cut out a strip of corrugated cardboard 14½ inches long and 1¼ inches wide. Ease the strip of card into a curve by running it between your fingers. Find the middle of the strip, form a crease, and position the crease around the bottom point on the base. Tape into position at right angles to the base. Apply tape both inside and outside the box.

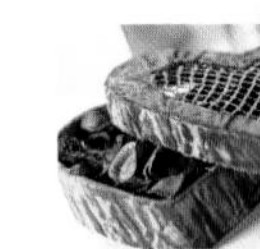

you will need

thick or corrugated cardboard

pencil

scissors

gold mesh or net ribbon

tape

orange velvet fabric

fabric glue

dewberry potpourri

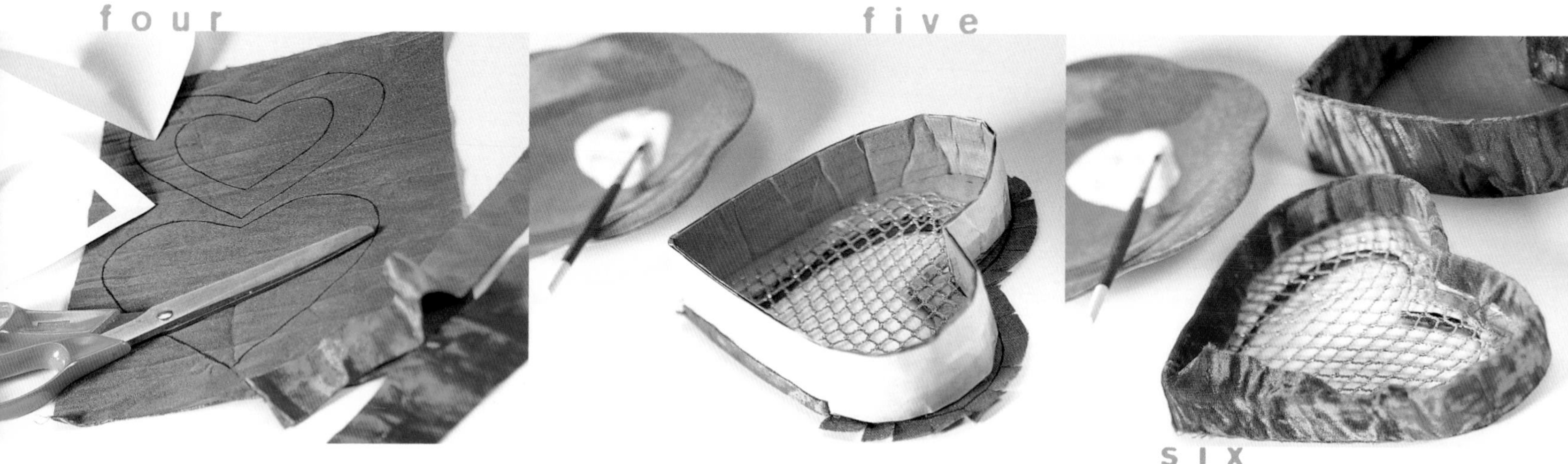

step 4 To cover the lid, find the tracing of the cut-out for the lid and make a template. Place it onto the wrong side of a piece of velvet and draw around it. Before cutting it out, allow a turnover of ½ inch around the outside edge. Repeat, but this time making no allowance for turnover.

Cut out a strip of velvet 18 inches long and 1 inch wide to cover the rim of the box.

For the base of the box, position the medium heart template onto the wrong side of the velvet, draw around it, and cut it out. Cut out a strip of velvet 14¼ inches long and 2½ inches wide to cover the side of the base.

step 5 Glue the velvet cut-out with the allowance onto the lid. With scissors, snip into the allowance, and glue the turnover to the side of the rim onto the side of the box. Work gradually around the lid.

step 6 Glue the strip of velvet around the rim of the lid, and while you work, fold the excess inside the lid, smoothing creases as you go, and glue into position. Glue the second cut-out piece of velvet inside the lid.

Cover the side of the base in the same way, then glue the remaining velvet heart onto the outside bottom of the box. There is no need to cover the inside of the base if you are using it for potpourri.

To finish, fill with dewberry potpourri and replace the lid.

AROMATIC GREETING CARDS

These collaged cards have been made using small pieces of papyrus, red rush, corrugated cardboard, and bark papers as backgrounds. The chiles, lavender, cinnamon, and peppermint add not only scent but also texture and color to these stylish ideas.

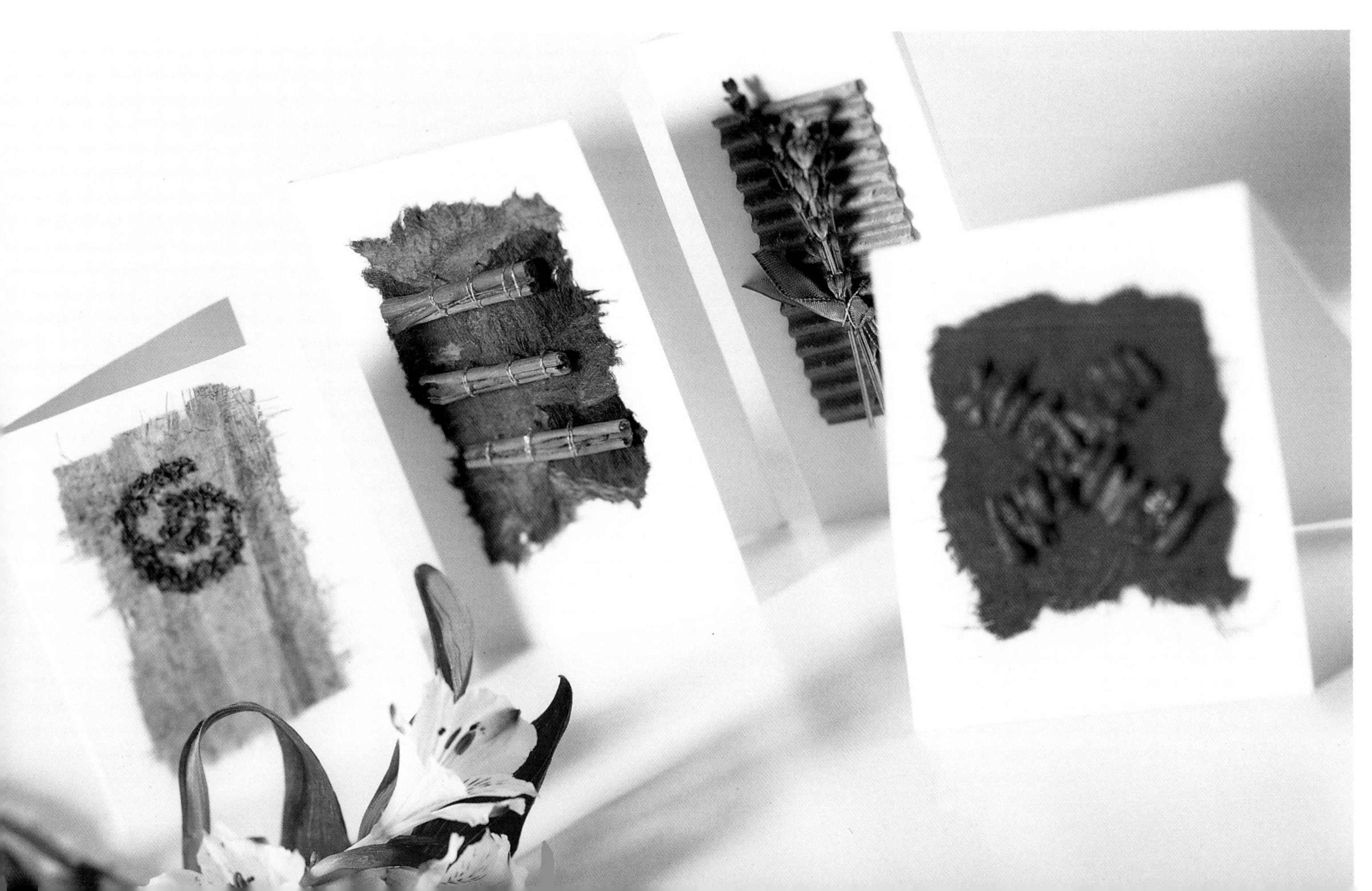

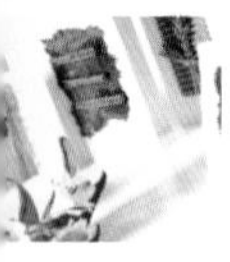

you will need

stiff white cardboard for the base cards

sheet of papyrus

sheet of red rush paper or other hand-made grass paper

corrugated cardboard

sheet of bark paper

pencil

white craft glue

wide brush

dried peppermint

small dried chiles

stems of dried lavender

ribbon

cinnamon stick

gold embroidery thread and needle

one

two

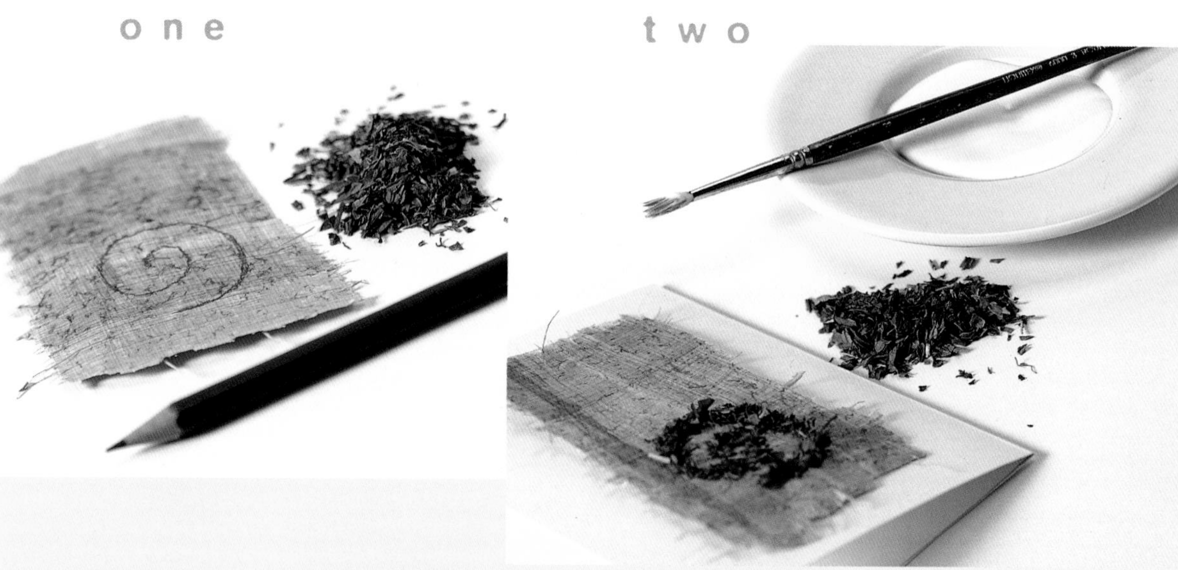

Folding the base card To fold stiff cardboard, it is necessary to locate the grain. You can do this by gently flexing the cardboard widthways, and then lengthways. Whichever exhibits the most flexibility determines the direction of the grain. Fold the cardboard along the grain to get a fold that is smooth.

papyrus and peppermint

step 1 Tear the papyrus to make a small square that will fit neatly onto the base card. Use a pencil to draw a swirl onto the papyrus. Apply glue to the pencil line.

step 2 Sprinkle dried peppermint onto the glue. Shake off the excess to reveal the swirl. Glue the papyrus to the base card.

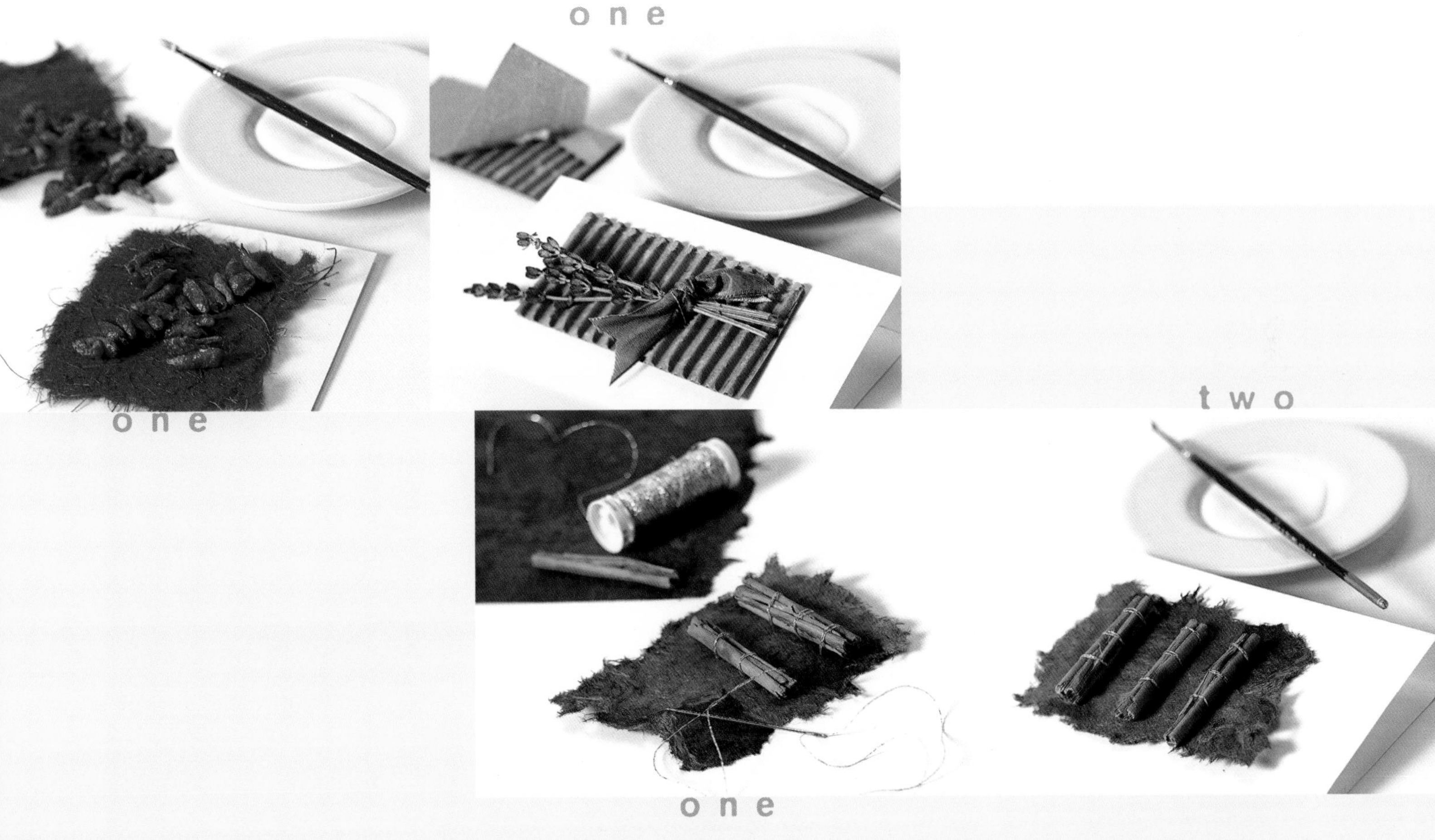

rush paper and chiles

step 1 Tear red rush paper into a shape that will fit onto the base card. Paint an X on the paper with glue and a wide brush. Position the chiles onto the glue. Let dry. When dry, glue the rush paper onto the base card.

corrugated cardboard and lavender

step 1 Cut a rectangle of corrugated cardboard and tear away the smooth outer layer to reveal the corrugated surface. Tie a bunch of dried lavender with ribbon. Sew the lavender onto the corrugated cardboard. Glue the corrugated cardboard onto the base card.

bark paper and cinnamon

step 1 Tear the bark paper to form a rectangle that will fit onto the base card. Break a cinnamon stick into three equal pieces and attach them to the bark paper using gold embroidery thread and a needle.

step 2 Glue the bark paper onto the base card.

CHAMOMILE BOOK COVER

An inexpensive note book or damaged hardback book can be transformed by covering it in cheesecloth and sprinkling chamomile flowers betweem the cover and the fabric. To give it as a gift, simply tie it with ribbon.

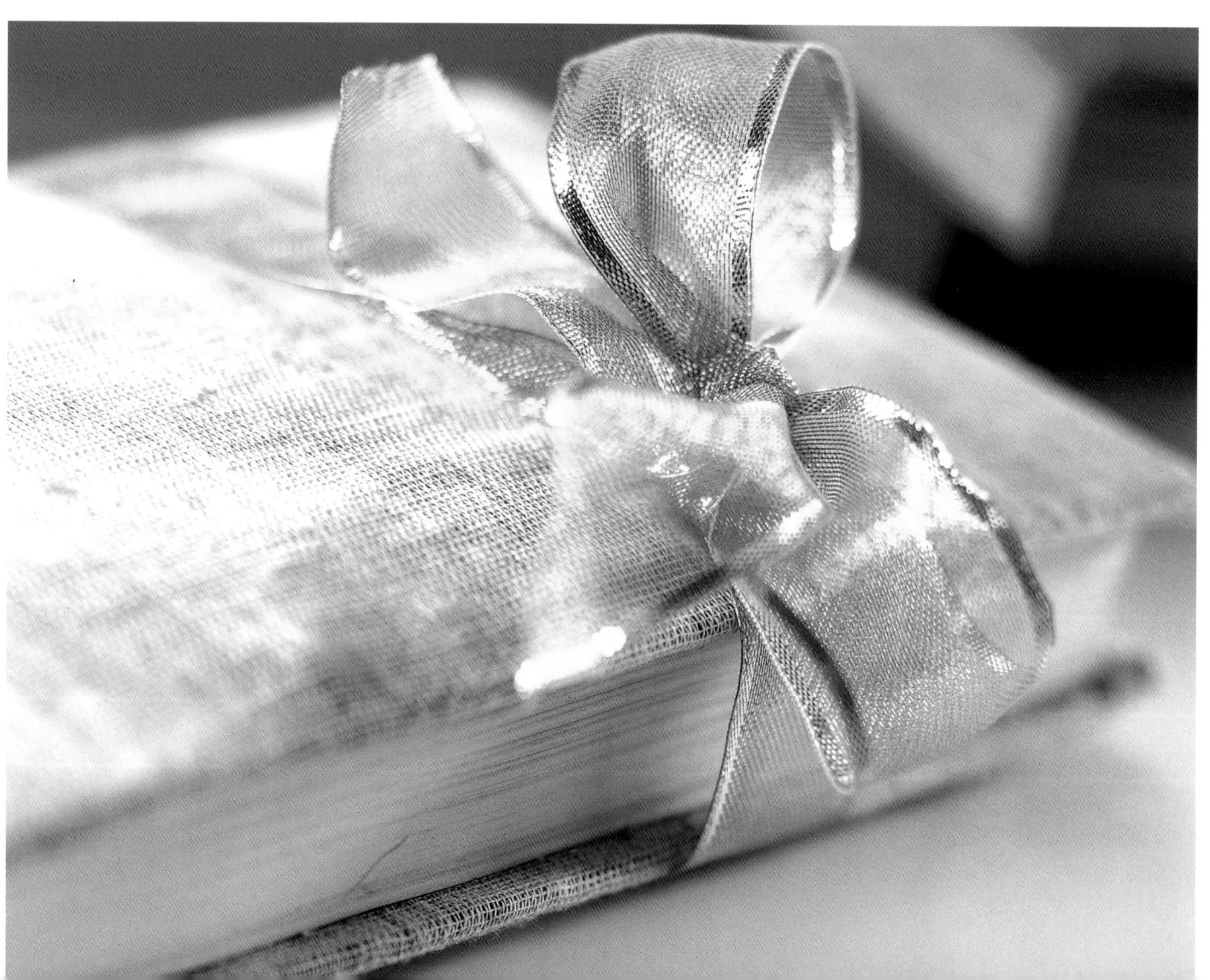

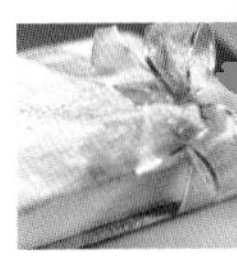

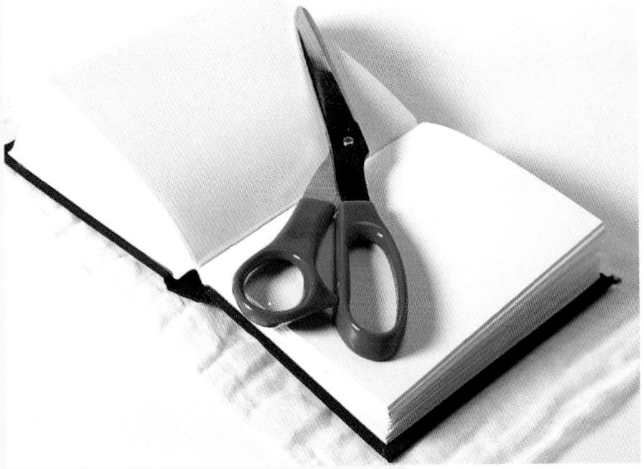

one

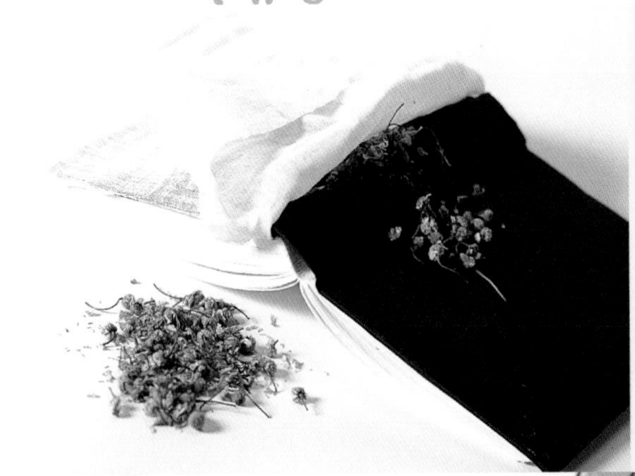

two

you will need

note book or hardback book

cheesecloth (butter muslin)

scissors

fabric glue

dried chamomile flowers

gold wired ribbon

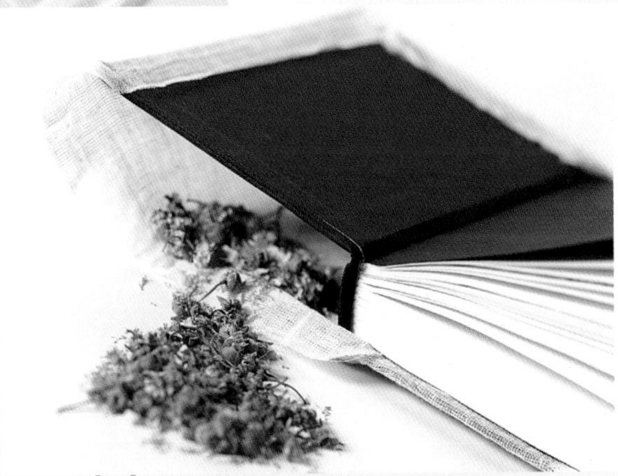

three

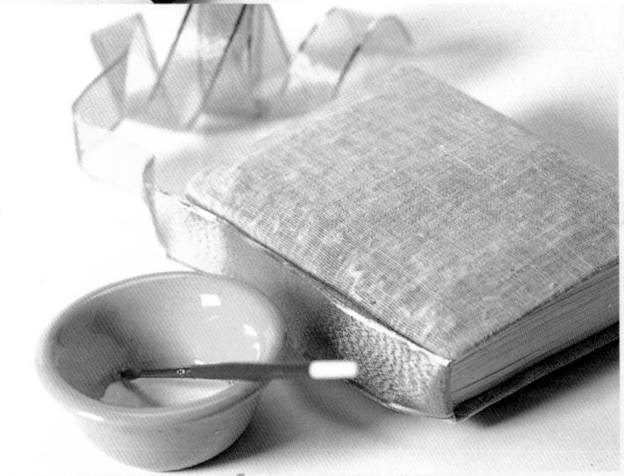

four

step 1 Place the open book onto the cheesecloth and cut the fabric to allow at least a 1-inch turnover along the top and bottom, and a 2-inch turnover on the sides.

step 2 Glue the turnovers into position on the inside cover of the book. When the glue is dry, place the book spine up, as shown, and sprinkle chamomile flowers into the pocket formed by the cheesecloth. Spread the flowers evenly and smoothly.

step 3 Lay the book spine down and pull the loose cheesecloth taut. Glue the turnovers along the top and bottom of the book. When dry, sprinkle in more chamomile flowers and smooth them out as before. Glue the remaining turnover.

step 4 Snip into the cheesecloth that is at the top and bottom of the spine. Apply glue to the snipped cheesecloth and push it inside the spine. Do this with the book open. Add ribbon to the spine in the same way. Close the book and tie with more gold wired ribbon.

VELVET PERFUME POUCHES

This soft and luxurious drawstring pouch is a wonderful and very practical alternative to gift-wrapping perfume. It's also reversible.

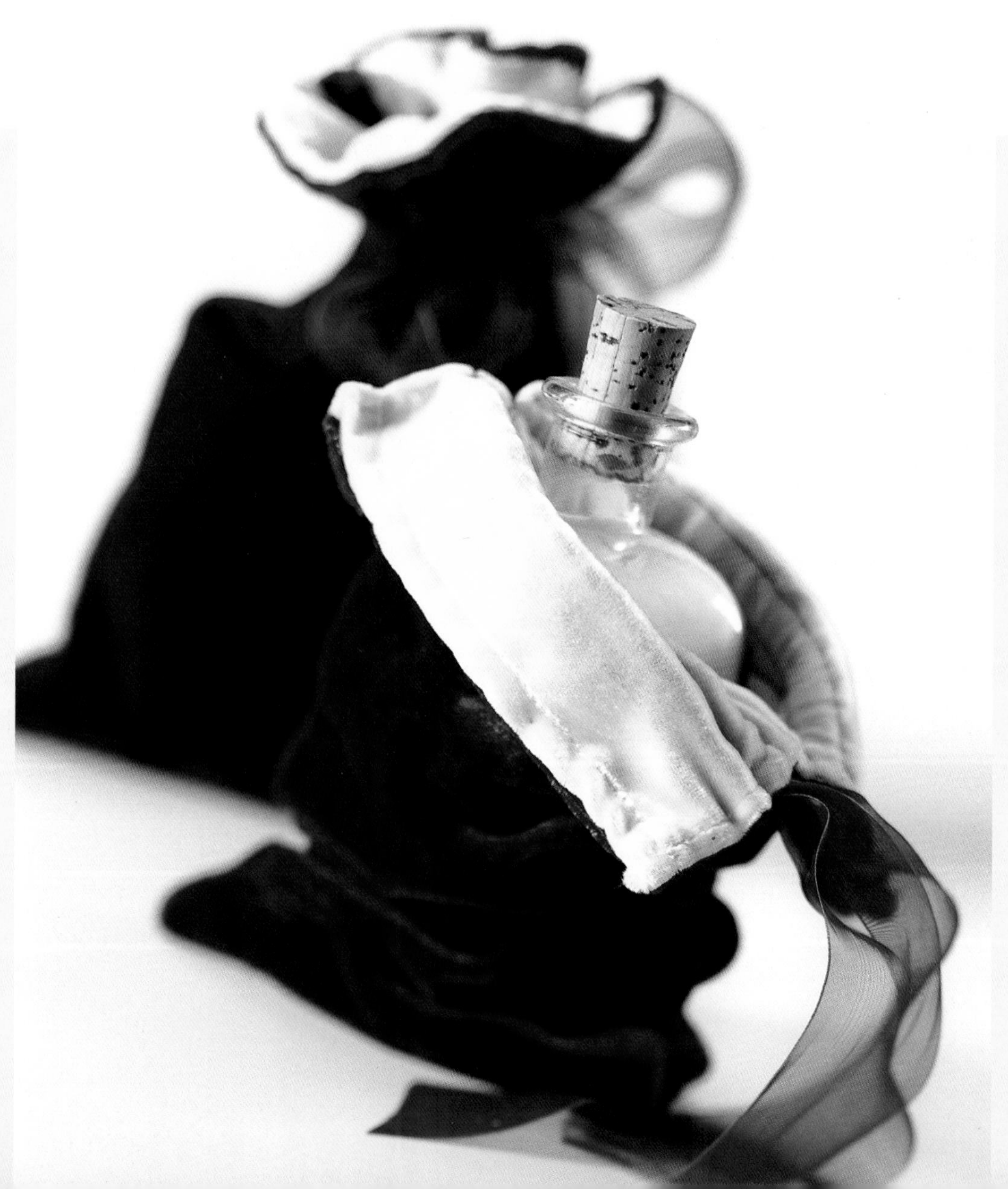

step 1 Cut 2 rectangles 20 inches long and 6 inches wide from both pieces of velvet. Stitch a small hem on all sides of both rectangles using the matching color thread.

step 2 Fold each rectangle in half, right sides facing, so that the folded fabric measures 10 inches by 6 inches. Machine or hand-stitch all the long sides, stopping 2 inches from the top opening.

step 3 Turn the blue velvet pouch right side out. Put the cream pouch, still wrong side out, inside the blue pouch. Pin the wrong sides together at the top open end and carefully hand-stitch them together with the navy blue thread using tiny invisible stitches.

step 4 To make a channel for the ribbon, machine stitch all the way around the pouch, keeping 2 inches from the top. Make a parallel line of stitches $\frac{1}{2}$-inch further down. Thread ribbon through the channels and pull tight to close the pouch.

one

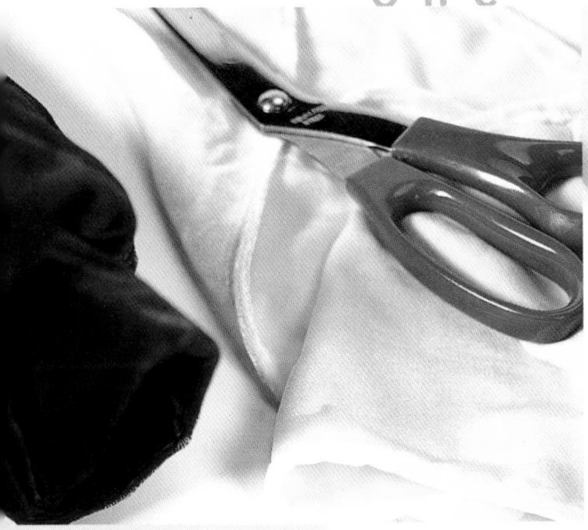

two

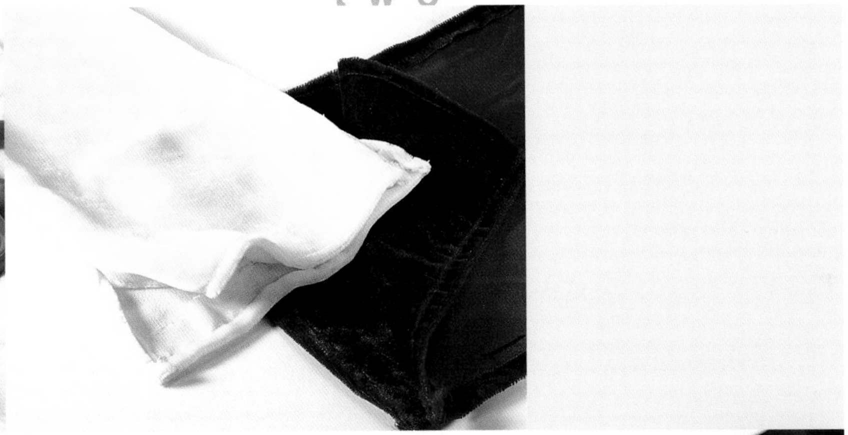

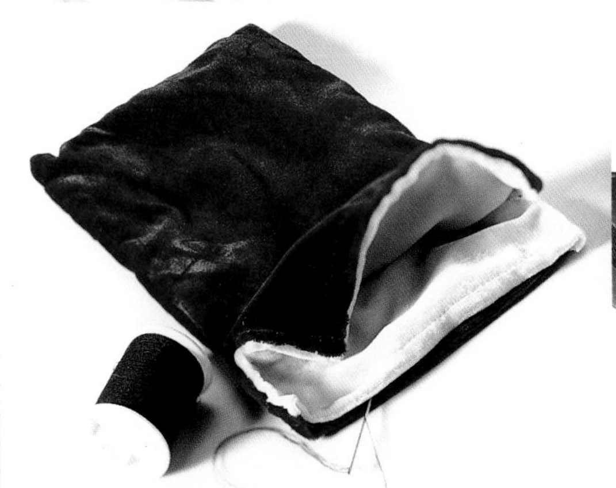

three

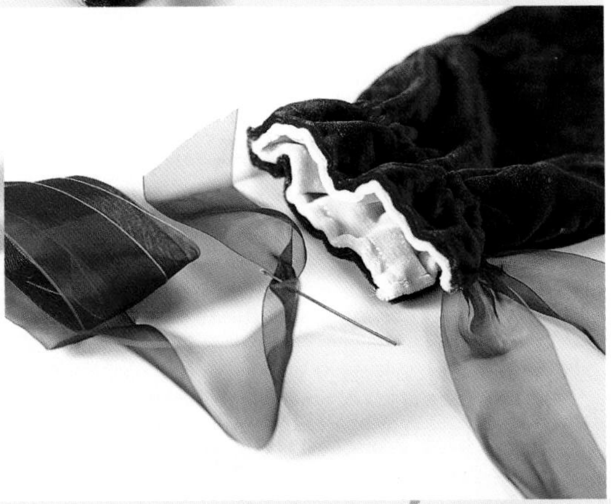

four

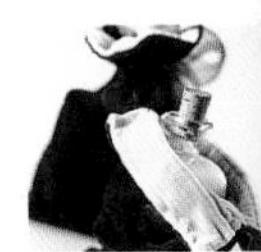

you will need

navy blue and cream colored velvet

tape measure

scissors

sewing machine

sewing needle

navy blue and cream sewing thread

sheer blue ribbon

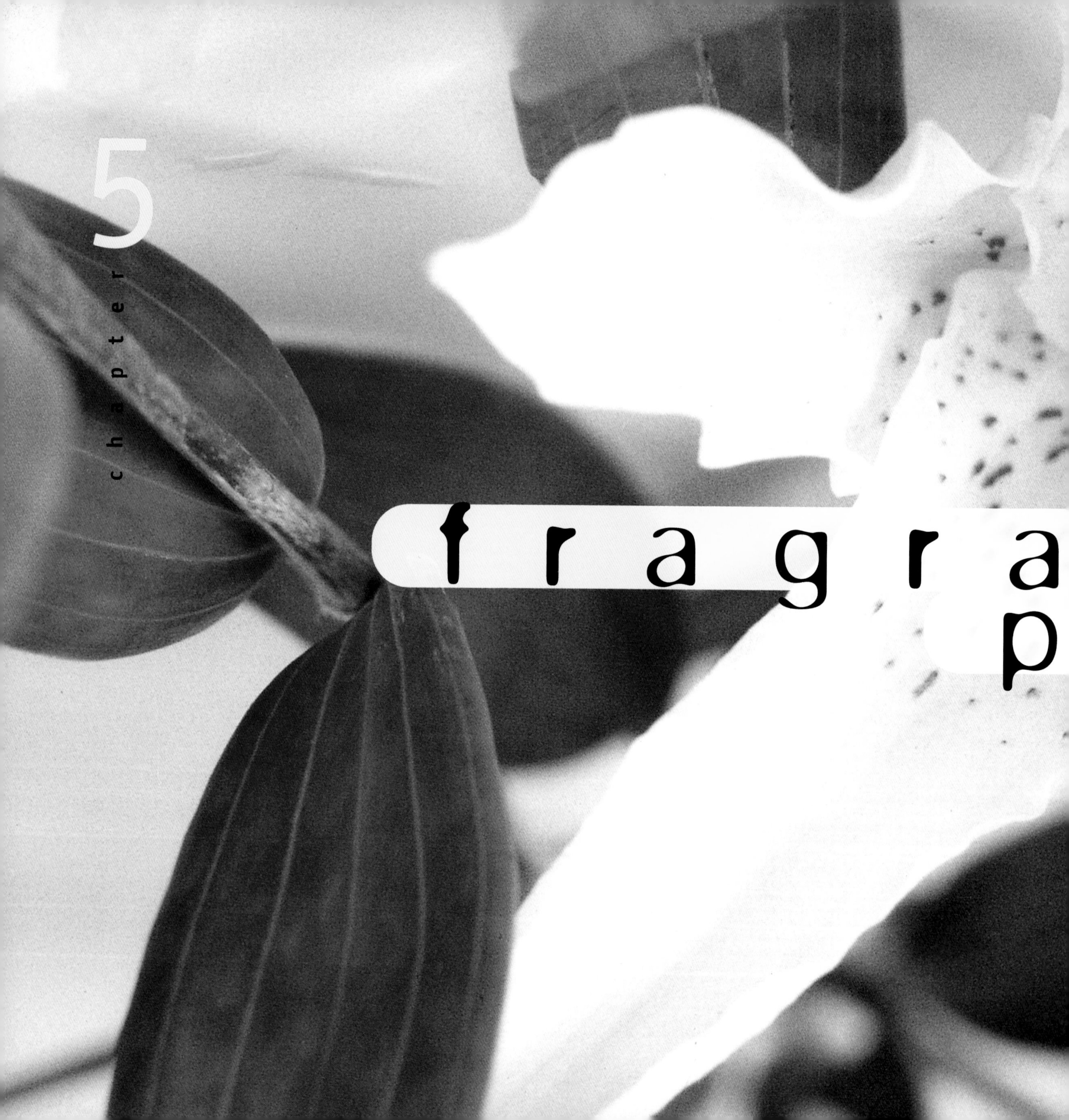

5

chapter

fragra
p

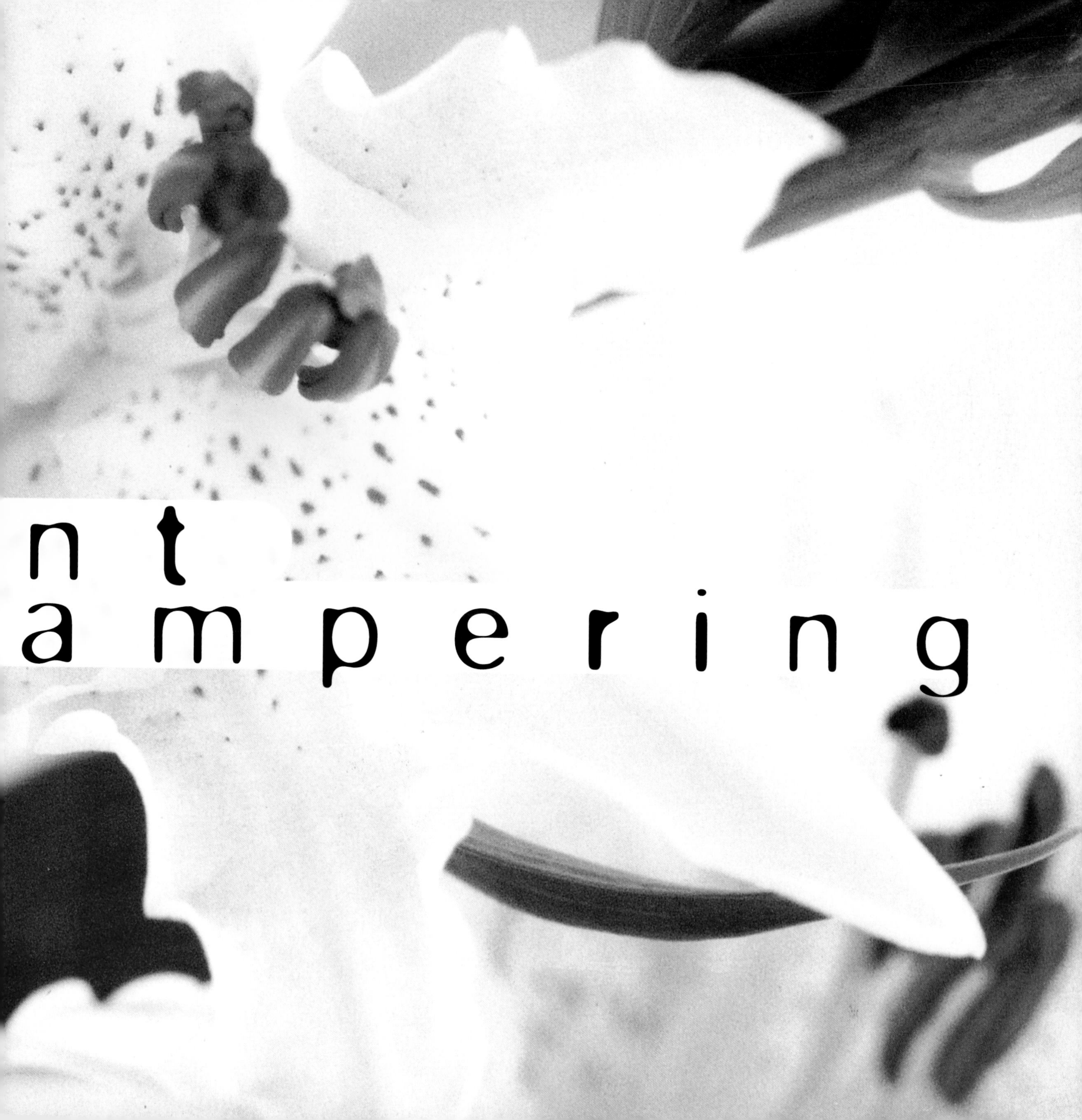
nt
ampering

ROSE AND SANDALWOOD CLEANSING FACE PACK

Rose water is especially good for the skin and has been used for many centuries in women's toilette. Smooth the cleansing and refreshing cream over your face and leave it in place for five minutes before gently wiping it off. Extra care should be taken with very sensitive skin.

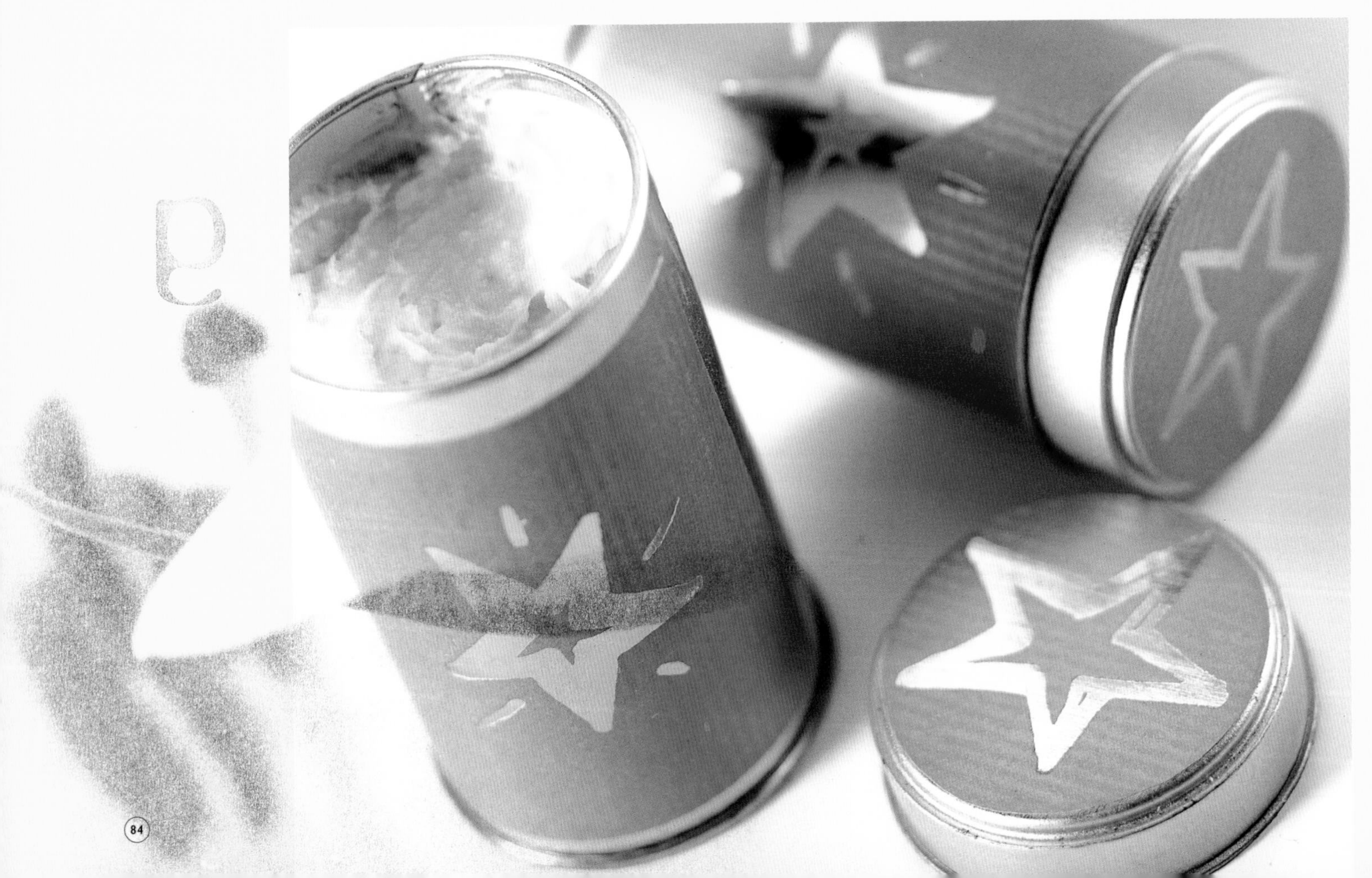

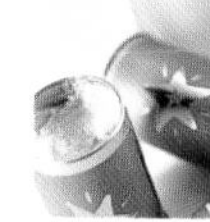

step 1 Mix the apricot kernel oil and the glycerine in a bowl over a saucepan of boiling water. Allow them to blend together and then set aside.

step 2 In another bowl, combine the lanolin and beeswax. Melt these ingredients together over the saucepan of boiling water.

step 3 Pour the kernel oil and glycerine mixture into the beeswax and lanolin mixture. Beat with a whisk until well combined.

you will need

scant 2 Tbsps apricot kernel oil

1 Tbsp glycerine

2 mixing bowls

saucepan

2 Tbsps lanolin

2 Tbsps beeswax

whisk

3 Tbsps rose water

large pinch of borax

sandalwood essential oil

one

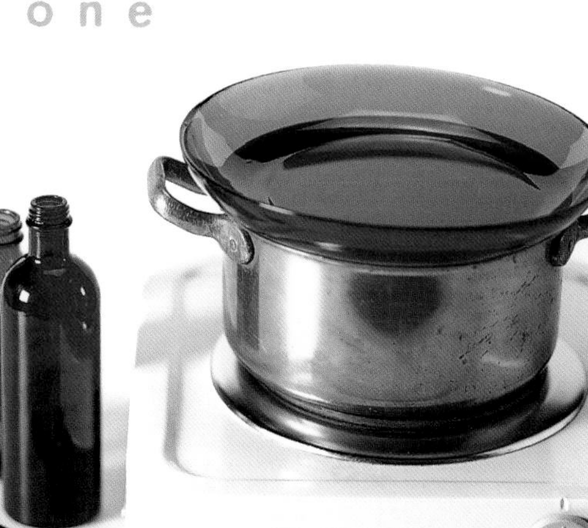

two

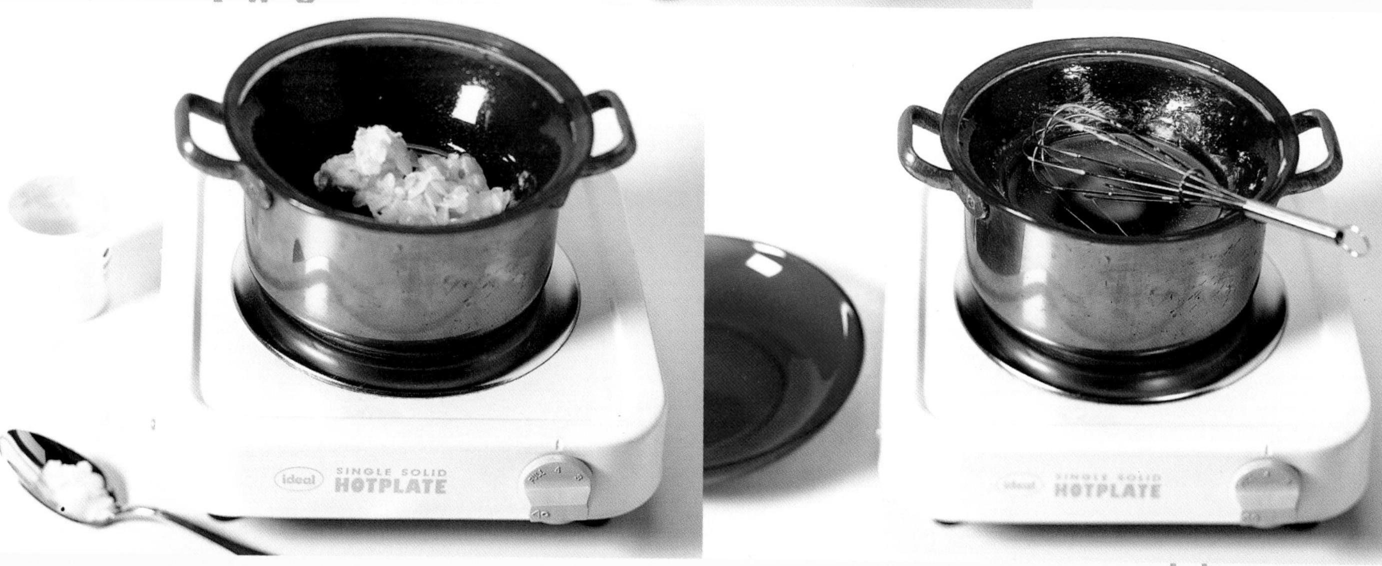

three

step 4 Gently heat the rose water and add the borax. When the borax has dissolved, add the kernel oil, glycerine, wax, and lanolin mixture. The texture of the resulting mixture will change immediately. Whisk to a creamy consistency. Remove from the heat and allow the mixture to cool for a few minutes.

step 5 Whisk the mixture to break down the skin that has formed on the surface. Continue whisking for 4 to 5 minutes to thicken the consistency. Stir in 3 to 4 drops of sandalwood essential oil.

step 6 Using patterns or motifs cut from a sheet of wrapping paper, decorate a plain, lidded container. Secure the pictures with glue, ensuring that they cover any existing labels.

step 7 Carefully spoon the scented cleansing face cream into the container and replace the lid.

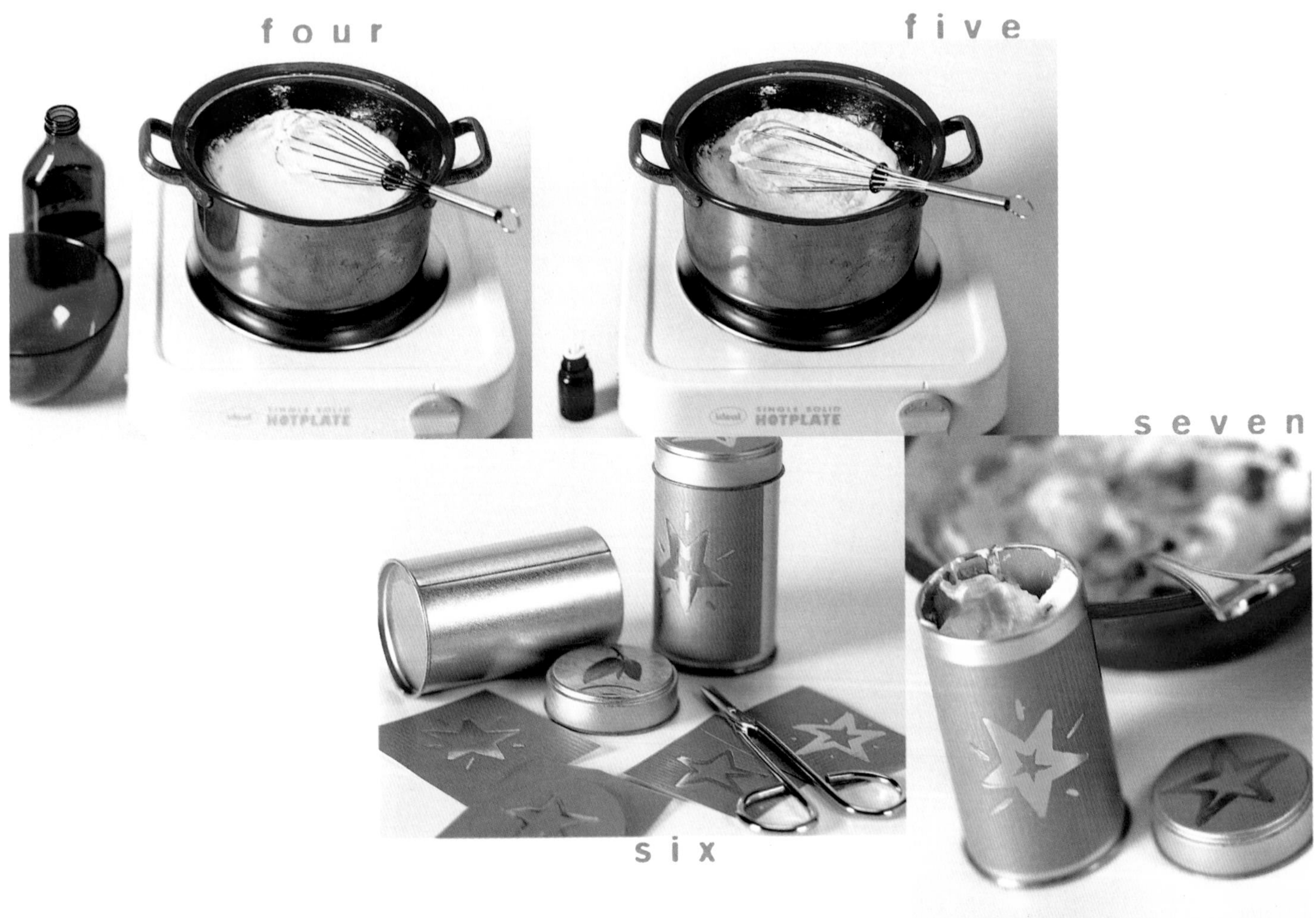

LEMON SOAP BALLS

So simple and inexpensive to make, these soap balls smell divine and look almost good enough to eat. It is worth knowing that a golf ball-sized soap can take up to two weeks to dry properly, so make them well in advance if you are planning to give them as a gift.

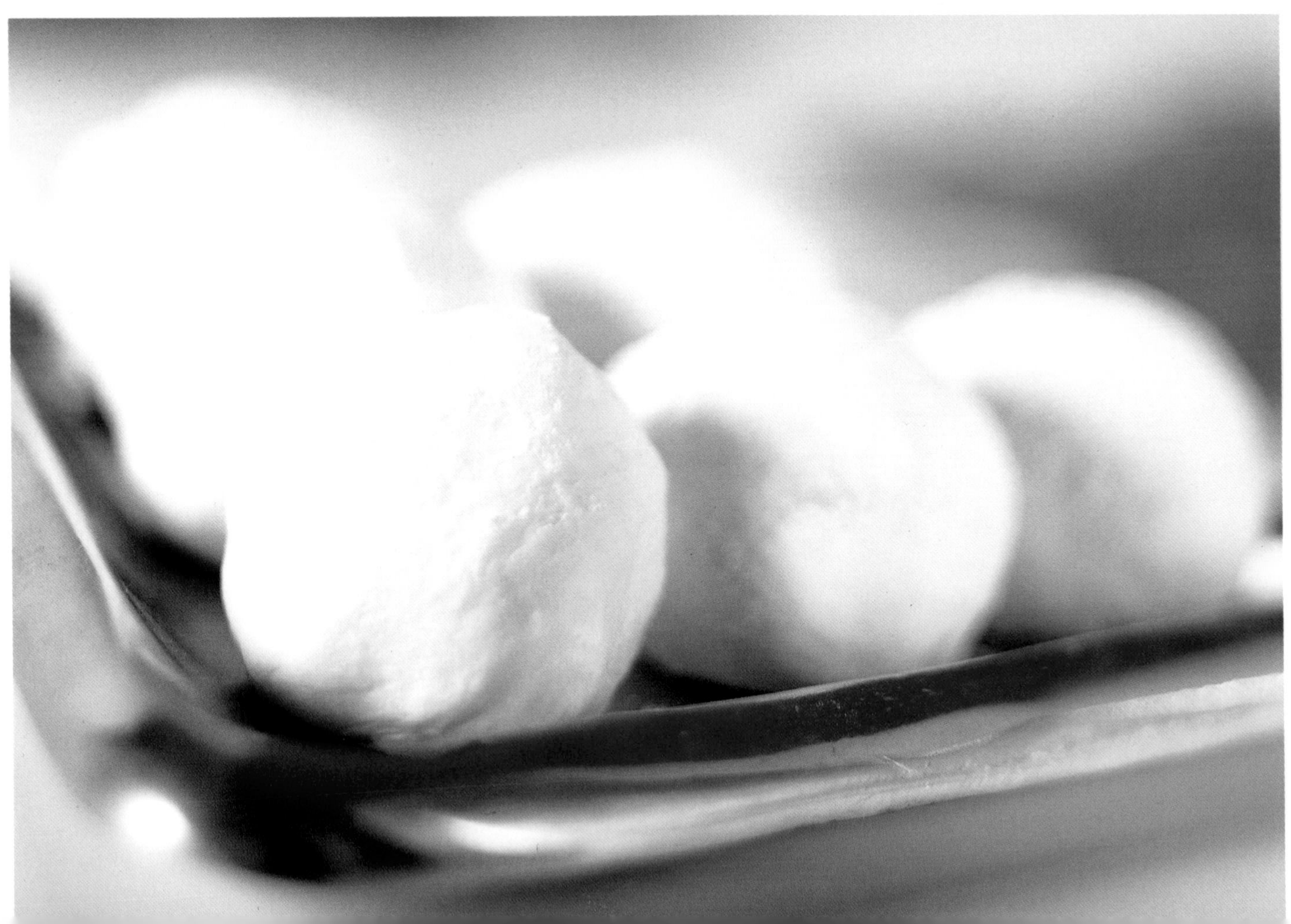

step 1 Finely grate the soap into a bowl. The finer the grated soap, the smoother the texture of the finished soap balls.

step 2 Add water to the grated soap in the ratio of 1 part water to 2 parts soap. Place the bowl over a saucepan of boiling water and mix together. Do not leave the mixture unattended, and stir continuously for 10 to 15 minutes until the ingredients are well combined and the mixture has the consistency of a thick paste.

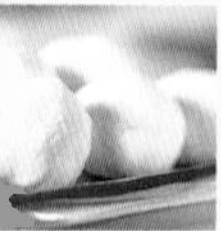

you will need

6 oz pure unscented soap

food grater

mixing bowl

saucepan

whisk

water

lemon essential oil

lemon-scented talcum powder

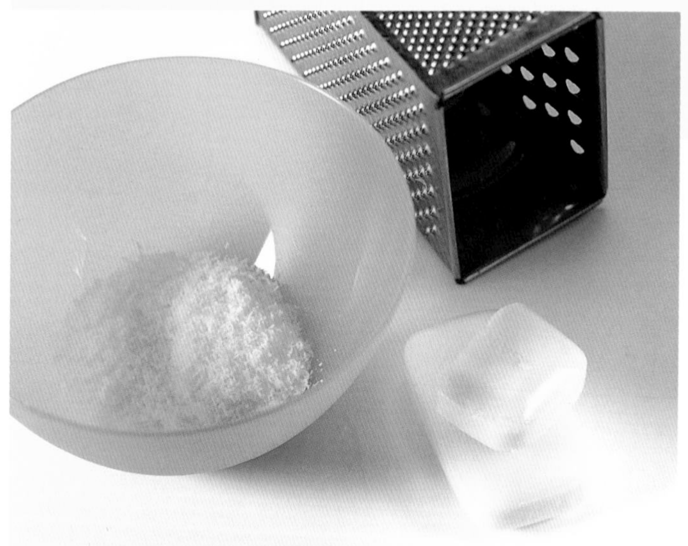

one

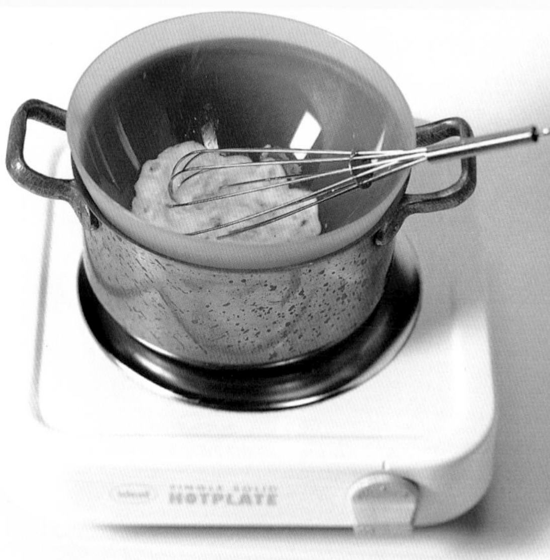

two

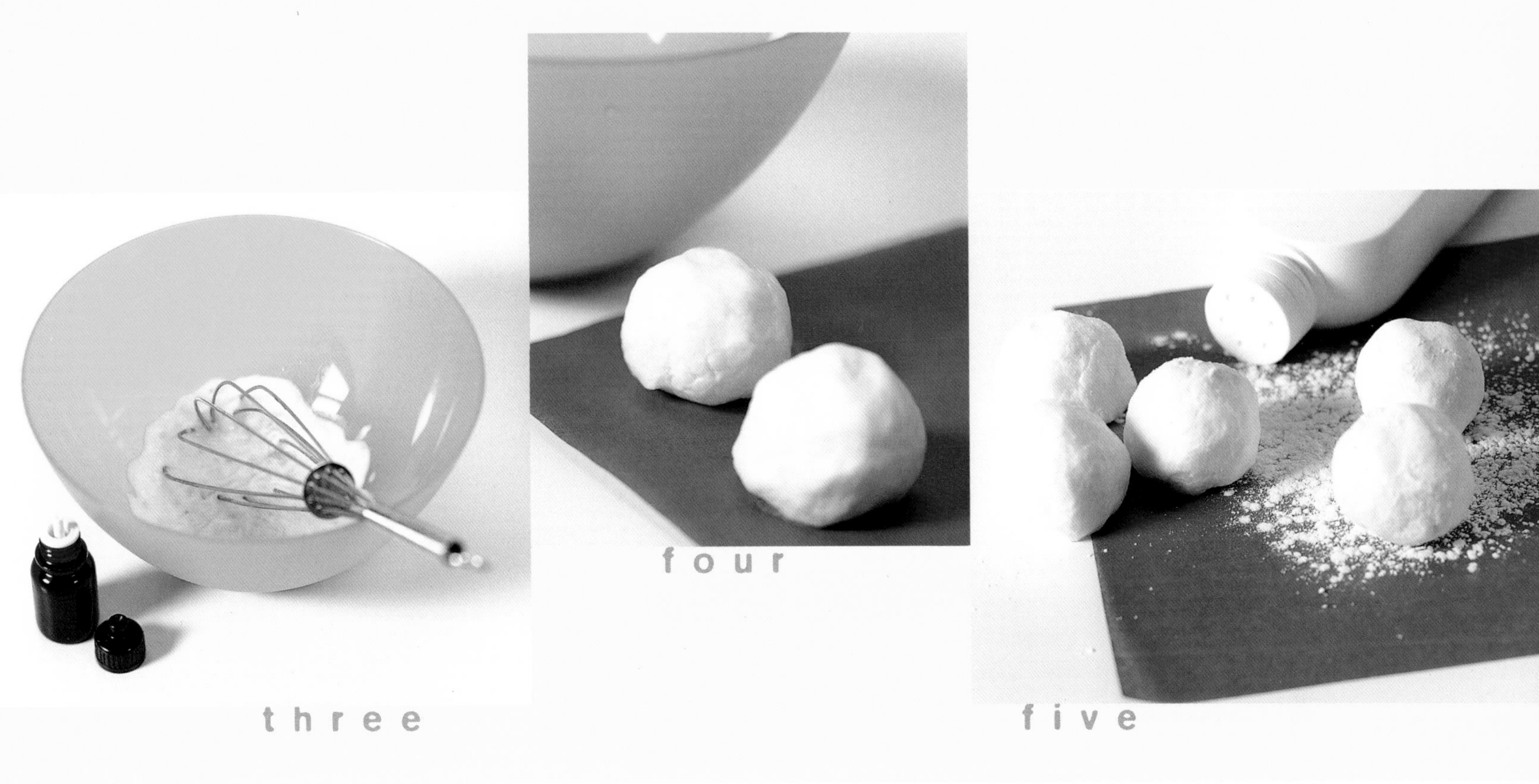

step 3 Remove from the heat and add 15 drops of lemon essential oil. Whisk the oil into the mixture thoroughly. Do not worry if the paste is rather wet.

step 4 Allow the mixture to cool for a couple of minutes and then dampen your hands with water. Take a small amount of soap mixture in your hands and roll it to make a ball. Place it on a plate. Repeat until all the mixture is used.

step 5 Leave the balls, which will still be quite sticky, to harden in a cool, dry place for about 4 days. Roll the soap balls in lemon-scented talcum powder and then set them aside for a further 2 to 3 days. When very dry to the touch, they are ready to use.

MIDNIGHT BLUE LAVENDER CUBES

These fun, velvet cubes can be used to scent drawers and wardrobes, or as playthings for a very special cat. Cats love the smell of lavender and find it reassuring and relaxing. However, do not decorate them with sequins or anything that a cat could swallow.

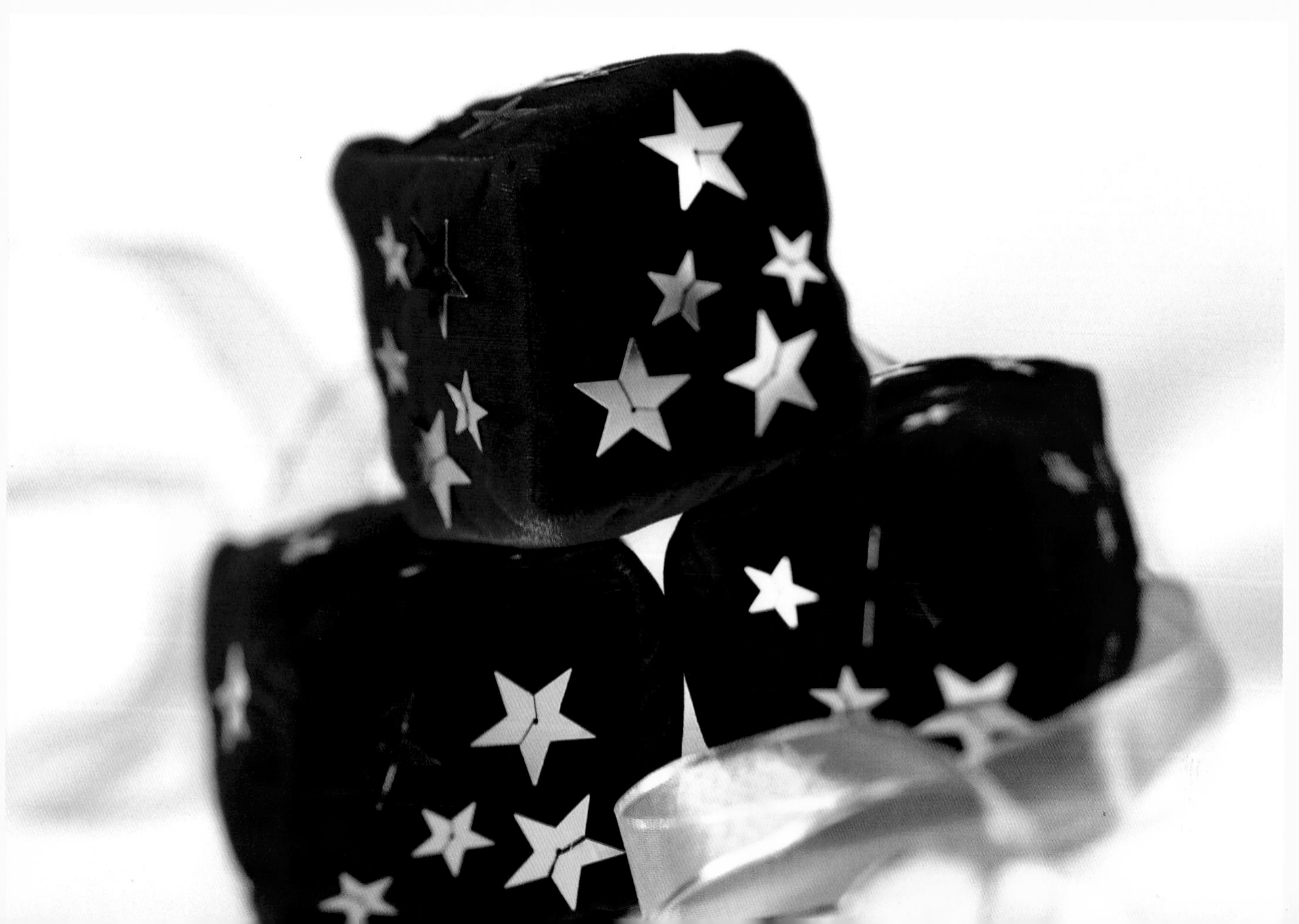

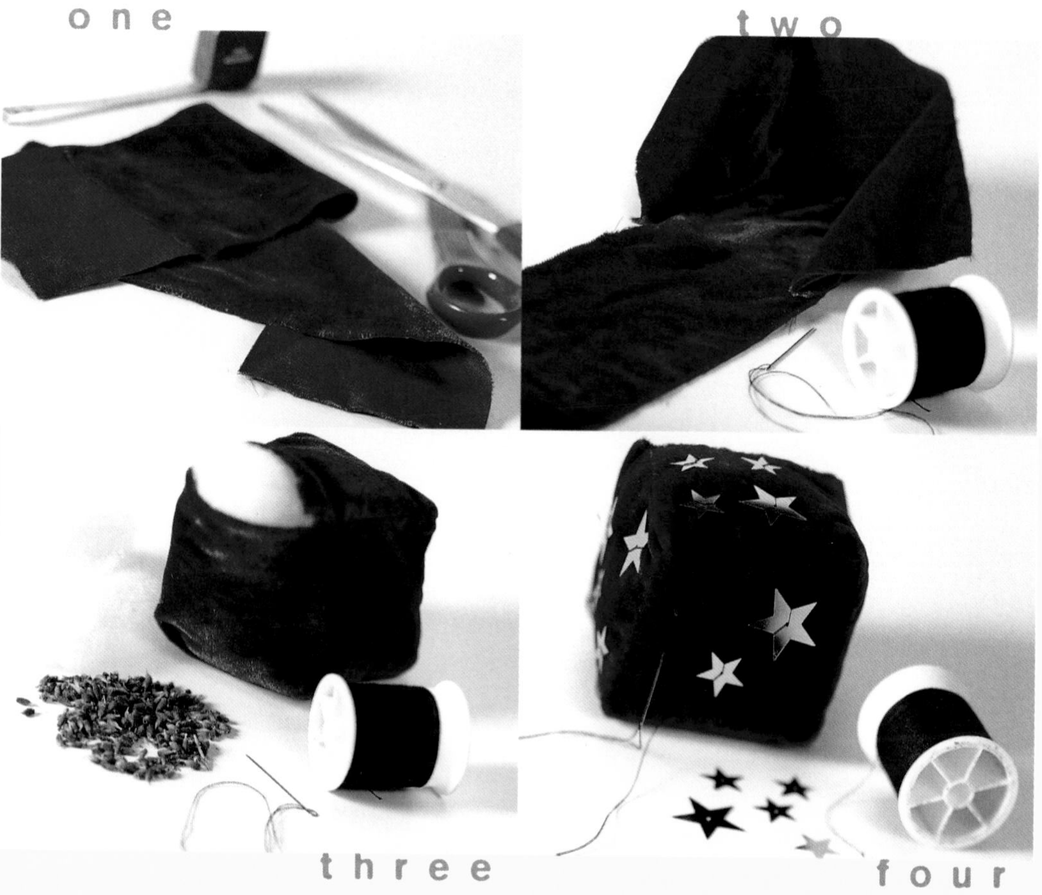

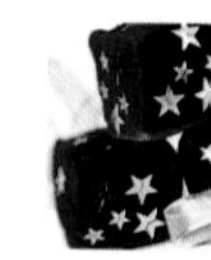

you will need

navy blue velvet

tape measure

scissors

fabric marker

dress-making pins

sewing machine

sewing needle

navy blue sewing thread

polyester batting (wadding)

dried lavender heads

gold star sequins

step 1 Cut two 9-inch by 3-inch rectangles of velvet. On the wrong side of the velvet use the tape measure to divide the long sides into 3-inch squares. Mark divisions with a fabric marker.

step 2 With right sides facing, position the strips of velvet to form a T-shape so that a 3-inch square of one strip covers the middle 3-inch square of the other. Pin together along the short end. Fold the strips to form a cube, facing in. Pin two more sides into position, and machine- or hand-sew the pinned edges together.

step 3 Continue pinning and sewing to form the cube, leaving an opening. Turn the cube right side out. Stuff the batting and dried lavender heads into the cube through the opening.

step 4 To finish, close the opening with hand-stitching and sew on the sequins.

VANILLA-SCENTED LIP BALM

The beauty of this lip balm is that you can make it in a couple of minutes using ingredients that you will find in your cupboard. Elevate this simple but effective lip balm by decanting it into a lovely old pill box or fancy candy tin.

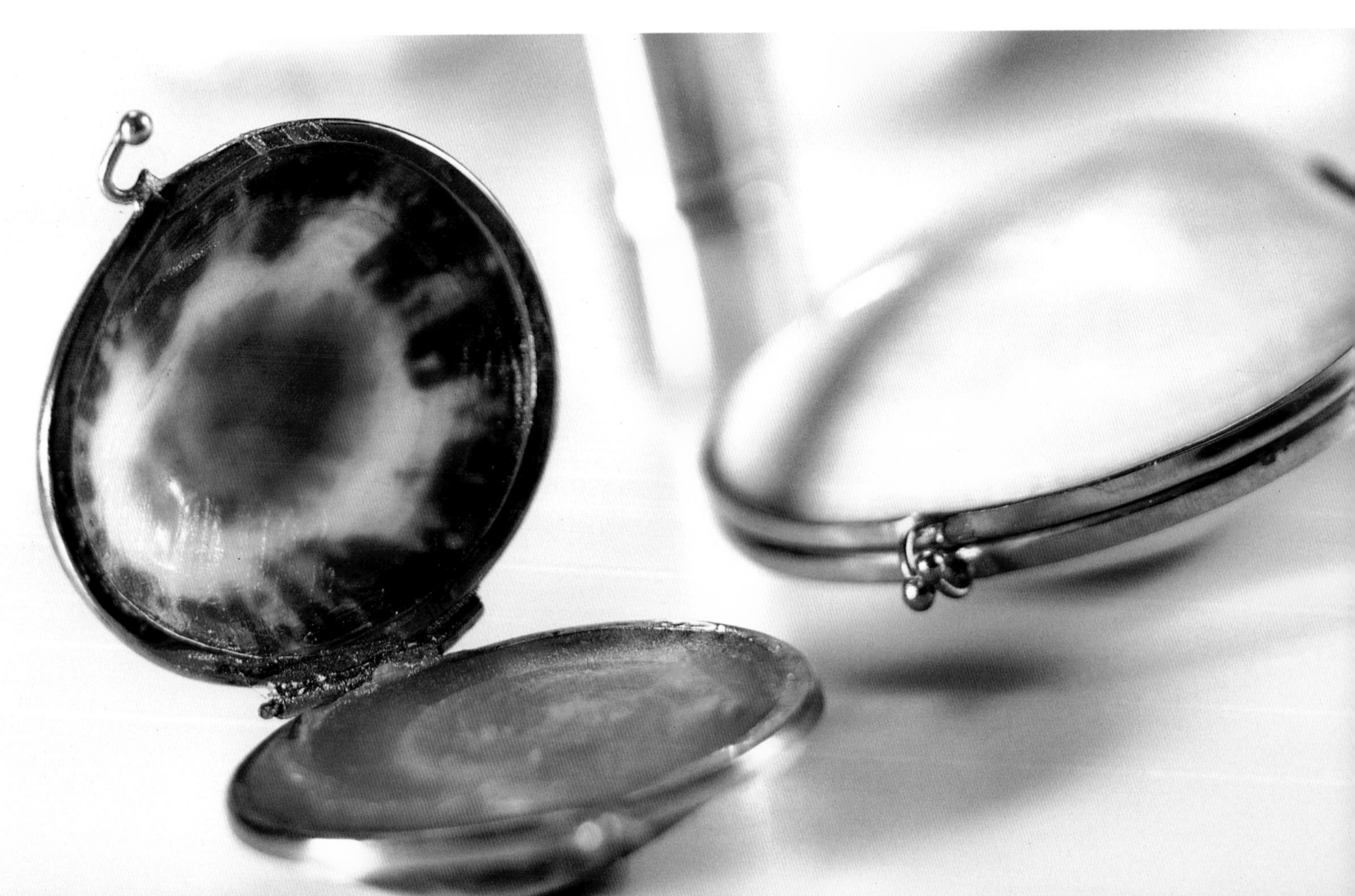

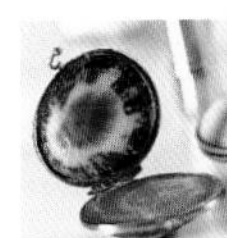

step 1 Mix together the petroleum jelly with the vanilla flavoring and blend thoroughly in a small bowl.

step 2 Add a sliver of terracotta lip color to the mixture. Blend thoroughly, ensuring that the color is dispersed evenly through the mixture. Squash unblended blobs of lip color with the back of the spoon.

step 3 Spoon into the container and your lip balm is ready to use.

you will need

3 tsps pure petroleum jelly

½ tsp of vanilla flavoring (essence)

small mixing bowl

spoon

terracotta lip color or lipstick

attractive container with lid

one

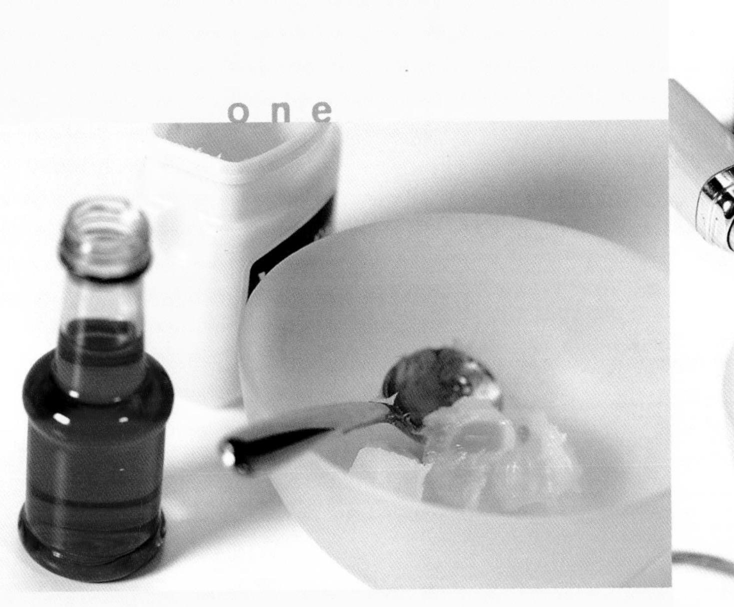

two

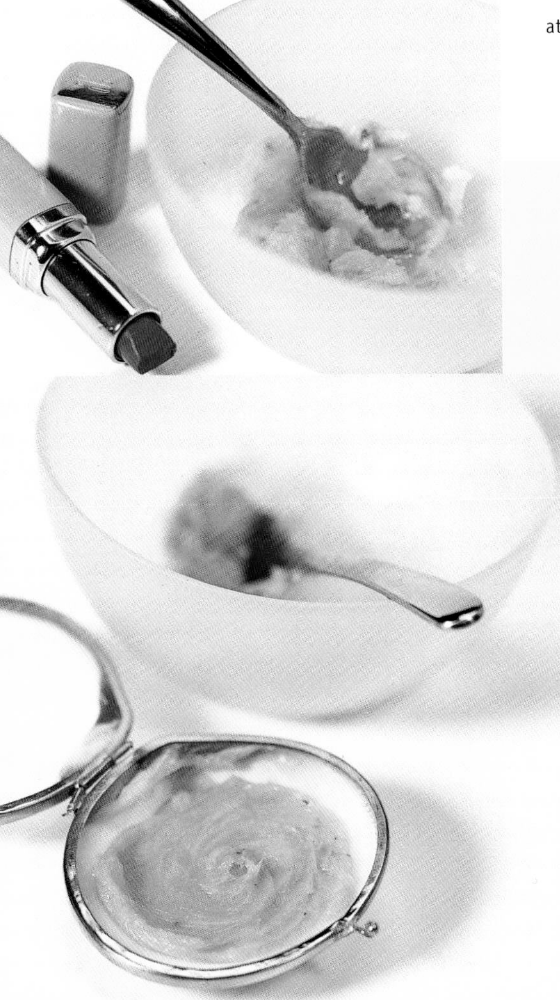

three

DEWBERRY SLEEP PILLOW

This scented pillow, which can be placed among your regular pillows, is perfect if you have trouble sleeping or simply want to enter slumberland on a cloud of beautiful fragrance. In place of dewberry, you can fill the pillow with dried chamomile flowers.

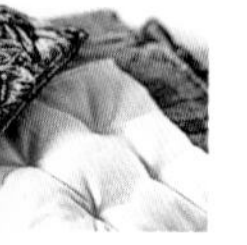

you will need

white cotton fabric

scissors

tape measure

sewing needle

sewing machine

white sewing thread

polyester batting (wadding)

piece of crushed velvet

dewberry potpourri or dried chamomile flowers

dressmaking pins

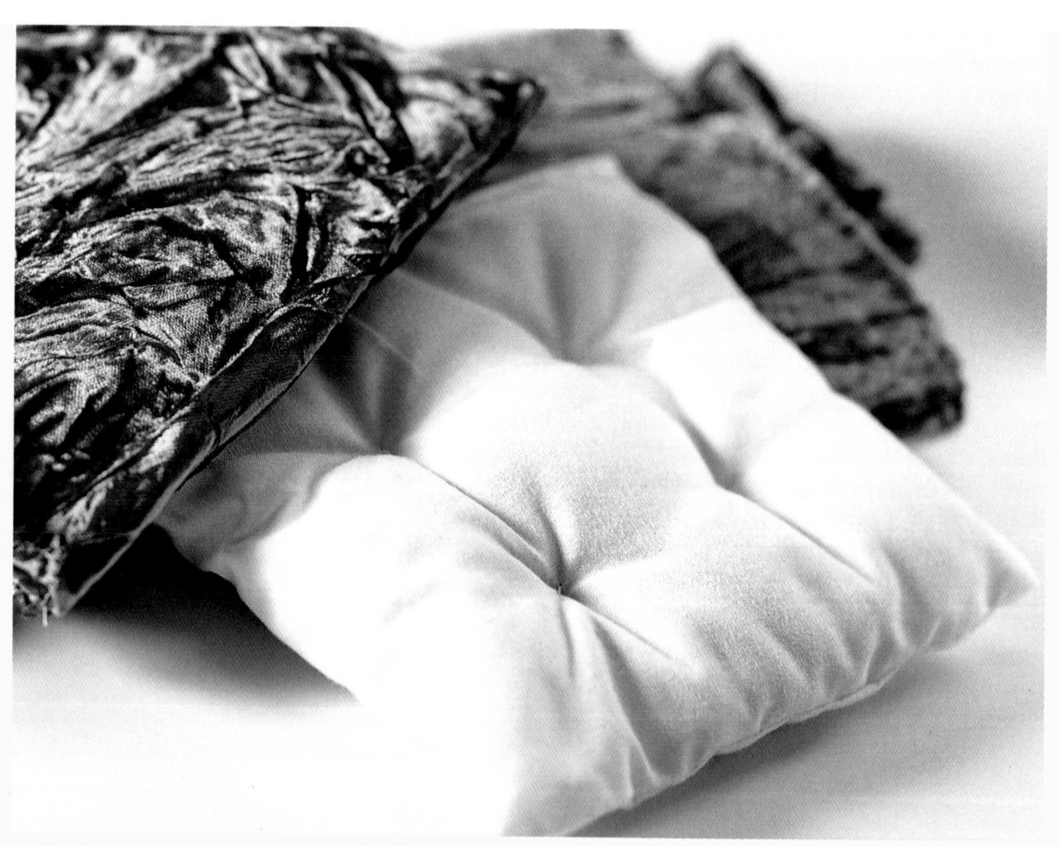

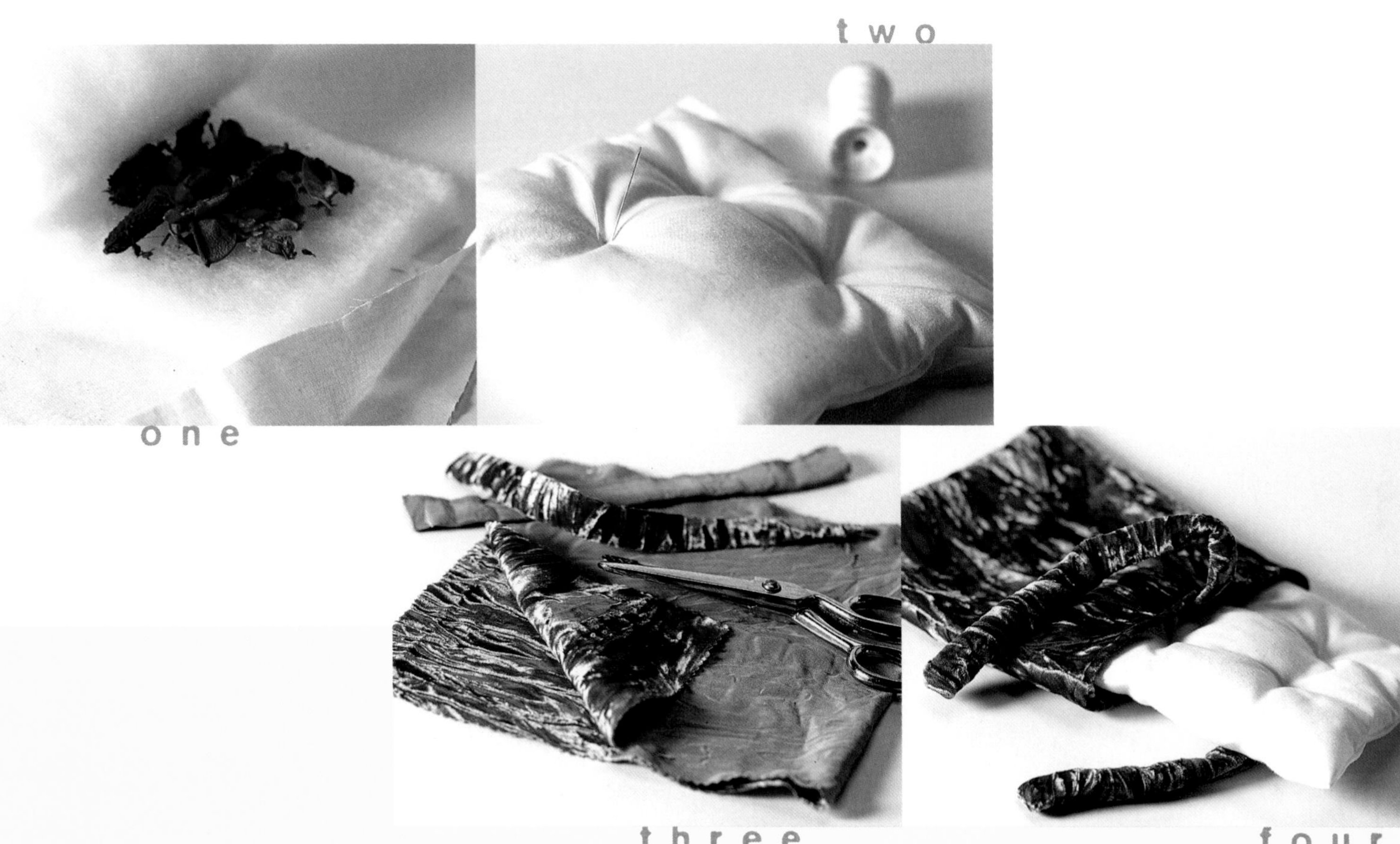

step 1 Cut a 16-inch by 6-inch rectangle of white cotton. Fold it in half lengthways and machine- or hand-sew up both sides, leaving the top open. Turn the pillowcase right side out. Cut a piece of batting 8 inches long and 6 inches wide. The batting should fit snugly inside the pillowcase. Pull apart the batting and sprinkle over the dewberry potpourri. Close up the batting.

step 2 Insert the batting into the pillowcase and close the opening with machine- or hand-sewing. To create the cushion effect, use a sewing needle and thread to sew four evenly spaced cross-stitches. The cross-stitches must catch both the front and back of the pillowcase.

step 3 Cut the velvet into a rectangle 16½ inches long and 7 inches wide. Fold it in half lengthways, right sides facing, and sew up both sides. Leave the top open. Cut two strips of velvet 7 inches long and 1½ inches wide. Fold them widthways, right sides facing, and sew along the length and one short side to make two straps. Turn them right side out.

step 4 Find the midpoint on both sides of the pillow cover opening and attach the raw edge of the straps with pins to the inside of the opening. The raw edges should be aligned. Turn over and hem the opening, catching the straps as you sew.

SCENTED BATH OILS

Commercially prepared aromatherapy bathing treatments can be quite expensive, but if you buy just one or two bottles of essential oils you can mix your own bath oils to suit your moods and needs. When bathing with essential oils do not use soap as it lessens the aromatherapeutic benefits.

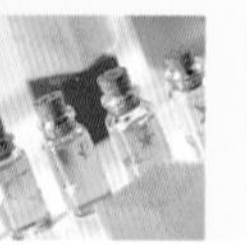

you will need

⅓ fl oz bottles with stoppers or caps

base dispersing bath oil

selection of essential oils

gold star stickers

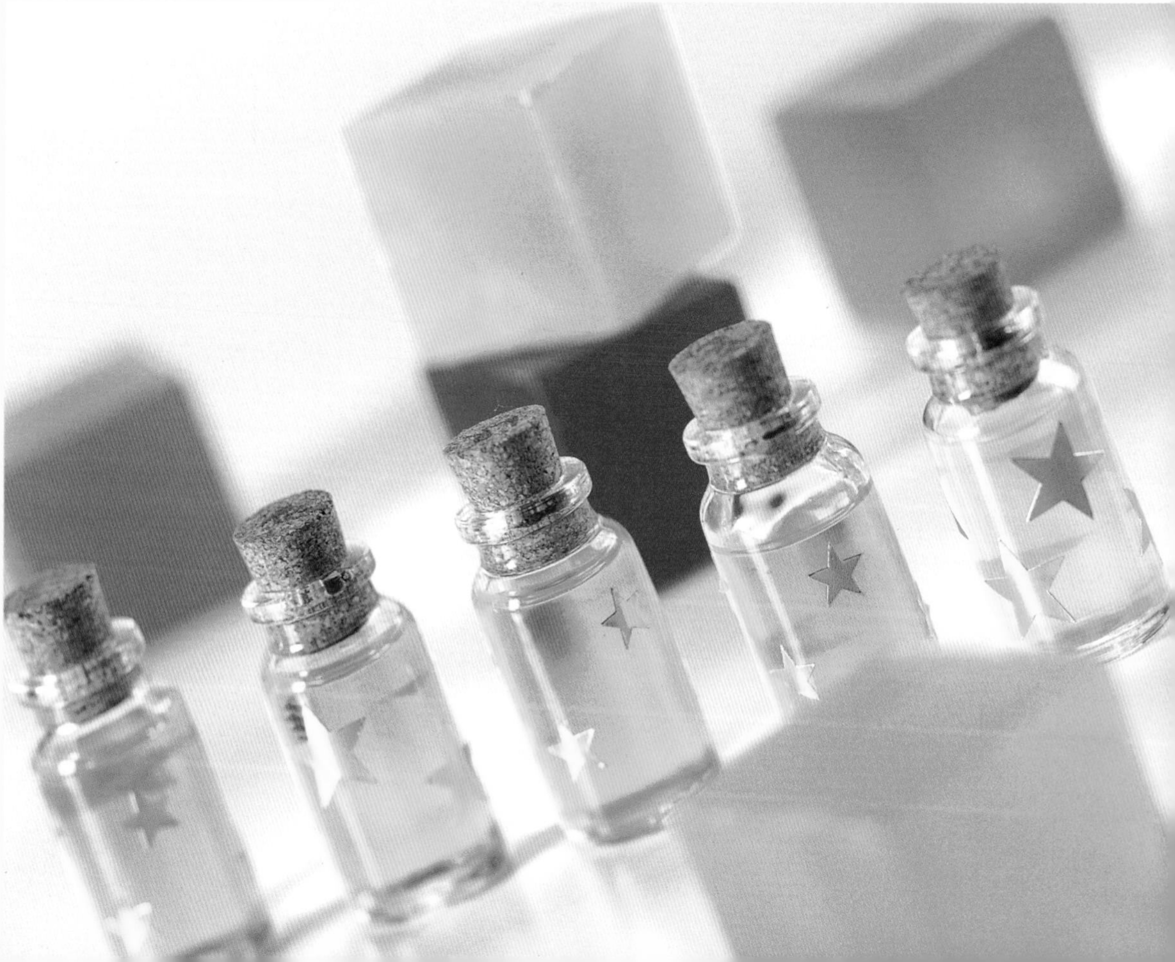

step 1 Fill the bottles almost to the top with the base dispersing bath oil.

step 2 Add the recommended amounts of the essential oils, replace the stopper or cap, and shake vigorously to mix the oils thoroughly.

step 3 Decorate the bottles with gold star stickers, and label and date each bottle.

one

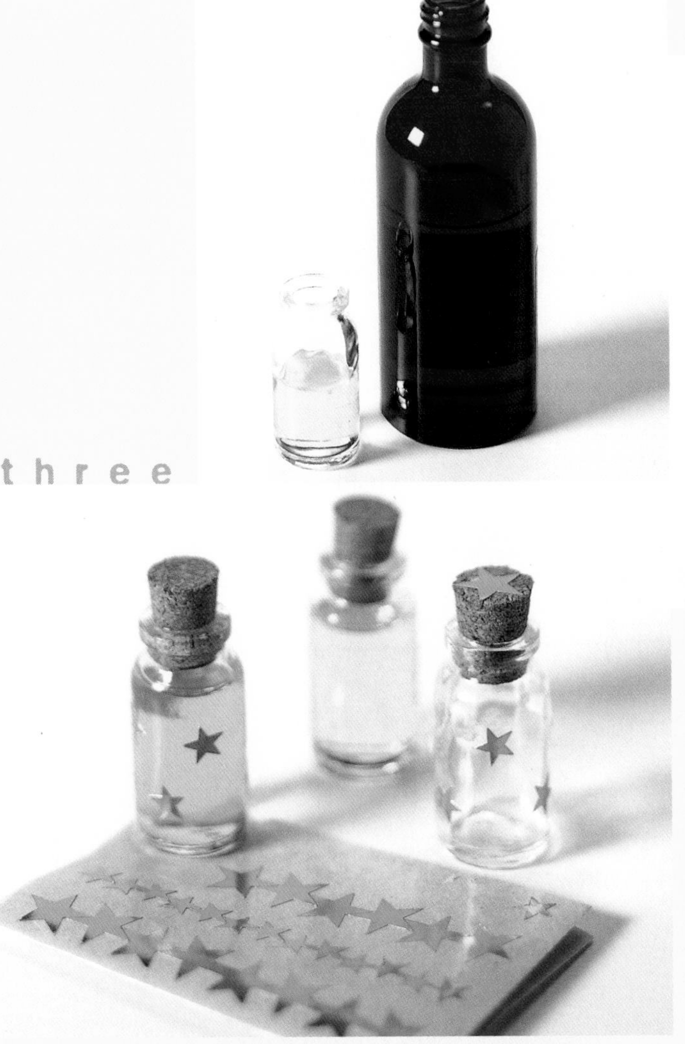

three

two

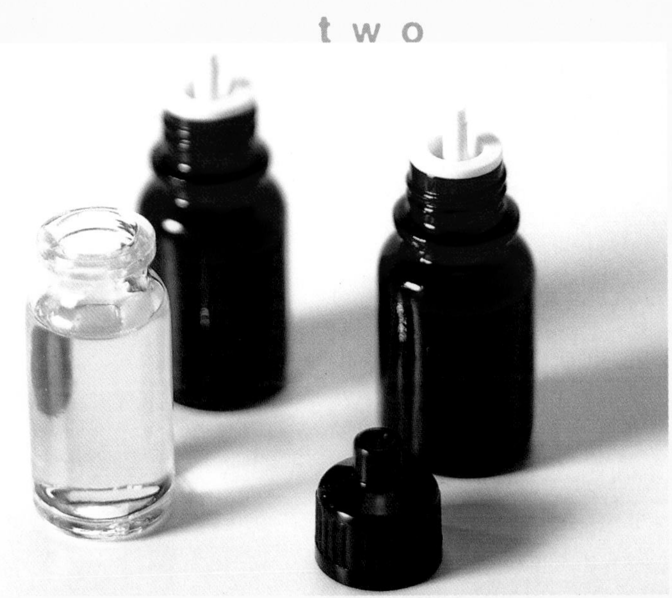

- **for cold and flu relief:** 2 drops eucalyptus and 3 drops lavender
- **for stress and overwork:** 2 drops clary sage and 3 drops lavender
- **for aches and pains:** 3 drops rosemary and 2 drops lavender
- **to counter Monday-morning blues:** 3 drops lemon and 2 drops rosemary
- **to stimulate the mind:** 1 drop peppermint, 2 drops rosemary, and 2 drops cedarwood
- **to relax:** 2 drops clary sage and 3 drops lavender

ROSE POT-POURRI

Many store-bought potpourri are overpowering with a synthetic scent. A home-made one using handfuls of dried rose petals and buds, essential oils, and a few basic ingredients is much subtler—its delightful fragrance almost unique.

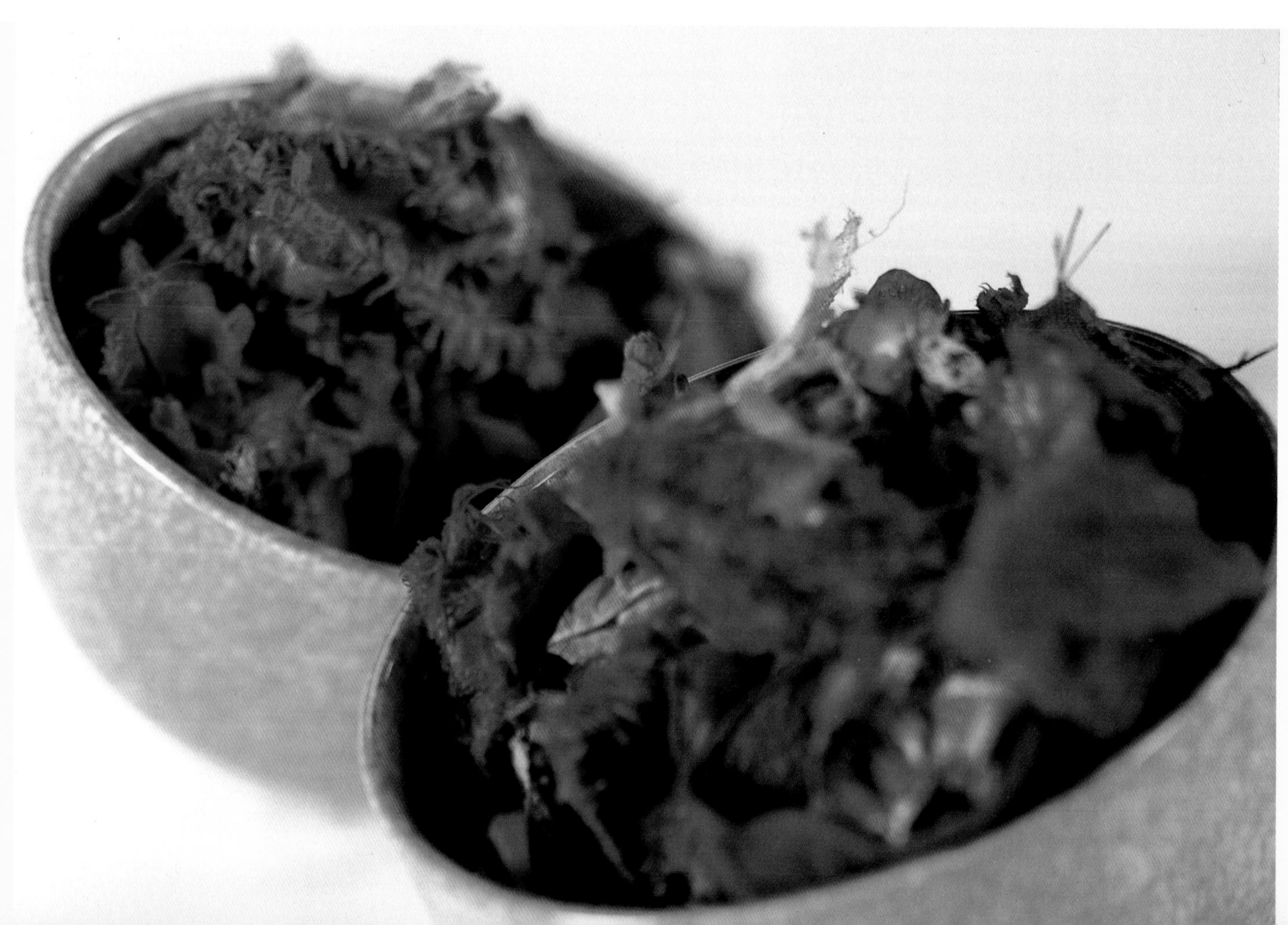

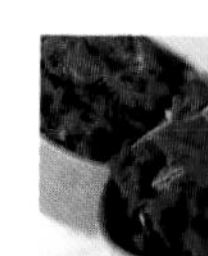

you will need

½ tsp bergamot essential oil

½ tsp lavender essential oil

¼ tsp geranium essential oil

½ tsp of clary sage essential oil

bottle with stopper or cap

6 tsps orris root powder

3 tsps gum benzoin tincture

pinch ground clove

pinch ground allspice

1 crushed cinnamon stick

small bowl

spoon

handful of dried red roses, petals, and buds

handful of dried pink carnations

handful of dried lavender flowers

handful of dried rose leaves

china dish

one

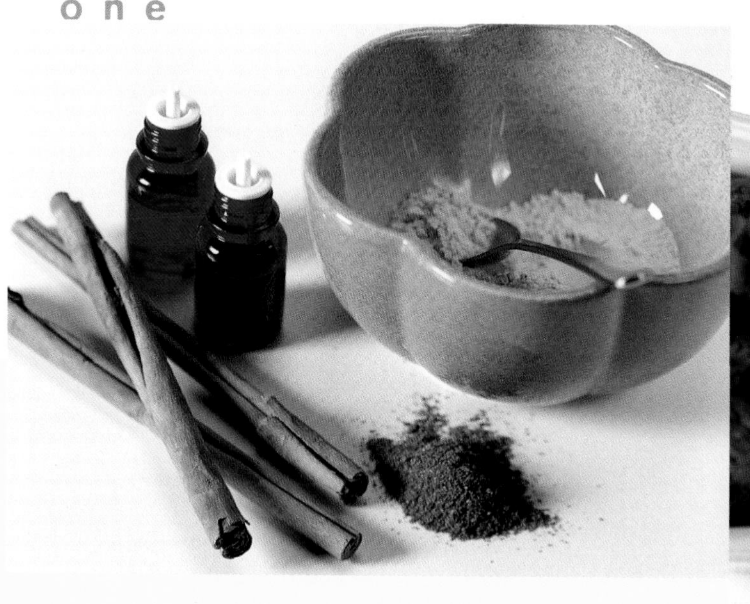

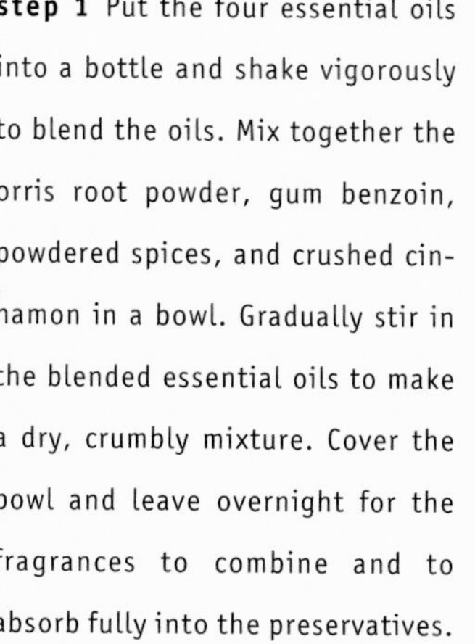

two

step 1 Put the four essential oils into a bottle and shake vigorously to blend the oils. Mix together the orris root powder, gum benzoin, powdered spices, and crushed cinnamon in a bowl. Gradually stir in the blended essential oils to make a dry, crumbly mixture. Cover the bowl and leave overnight for the fragrances to combine and to absorb fully into the preservatives.

step 2 Mix all the dried flower and leaf ingredients together in a china dish. Sprinkle on the oil, spice, and preservative mixture. Gently stir and agitate until the mixture is well dispersed. Cover and leave for two weeks in a warm, dry place to allow the fragrances to mature.

ROSE WATER TONIC

This rose water tonic is an ideal skin toner to invigorate and condition the skin after cleansing. Store this tonic in a cool place, out of direct sunlight. You should always label and date home-made cosmetics.

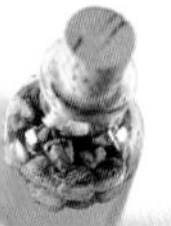

you will need

½ cup rose water

3 drops rose essential oil

1 tsp glycerine

4 Tbsps liquid witch hazel

screw-top jar

bottle, with stopper or cap, for storing the tonic

dried tiny rosebuds

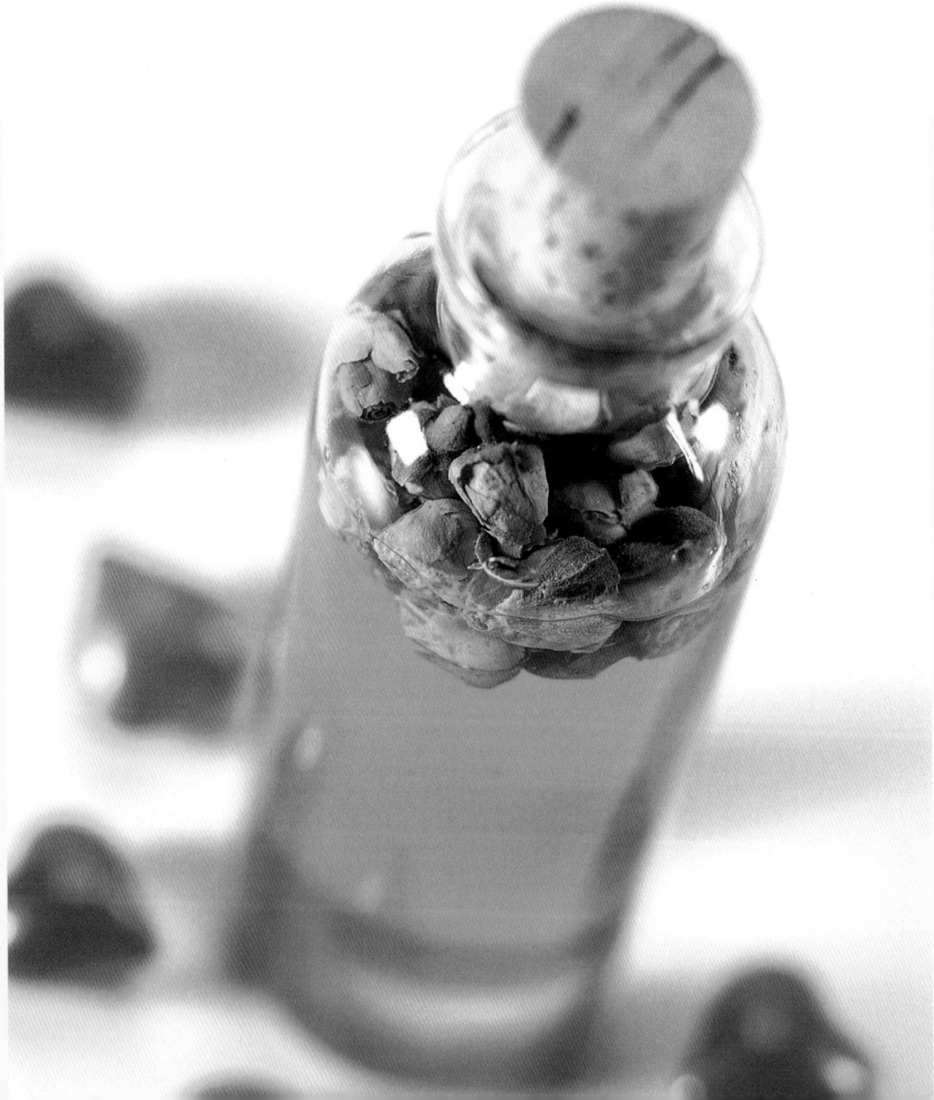

one

two

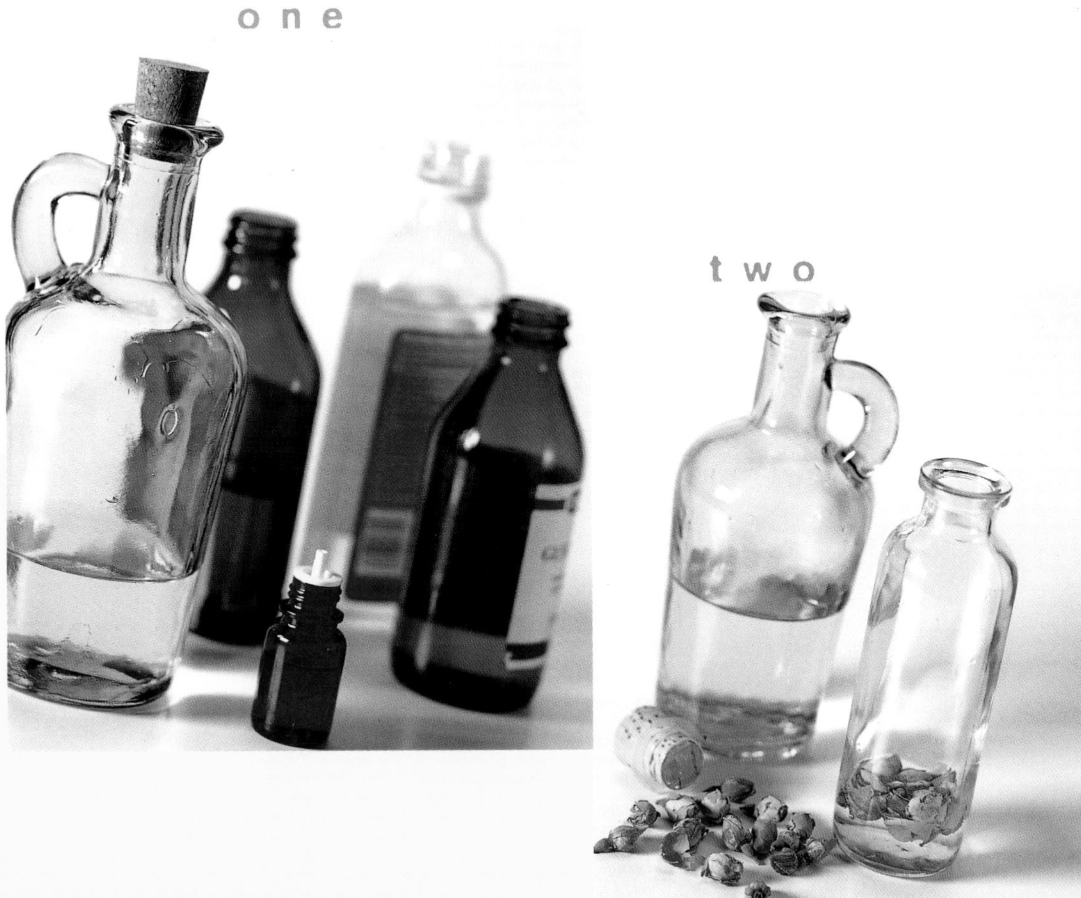

step 1 Put the rose water, essential oil, glycerine, and witch hazel into a screw-top jar, and shake vigorously to blend the liquids.

step 2 Put a small handful of dried rosebuds into the bottle. Pour in the rose water mixture and replace the stopper. The rosebuds will float to the surface.

SCENTED BODY LOTIONS

After bathing in your own aromatherapy bath oils, why not heighten the benefits by using the same oils in a rich body lotion. Massage the lotion into your skin in a circular motion. This will help to stimulate the skin and increase its absorption of the oils.

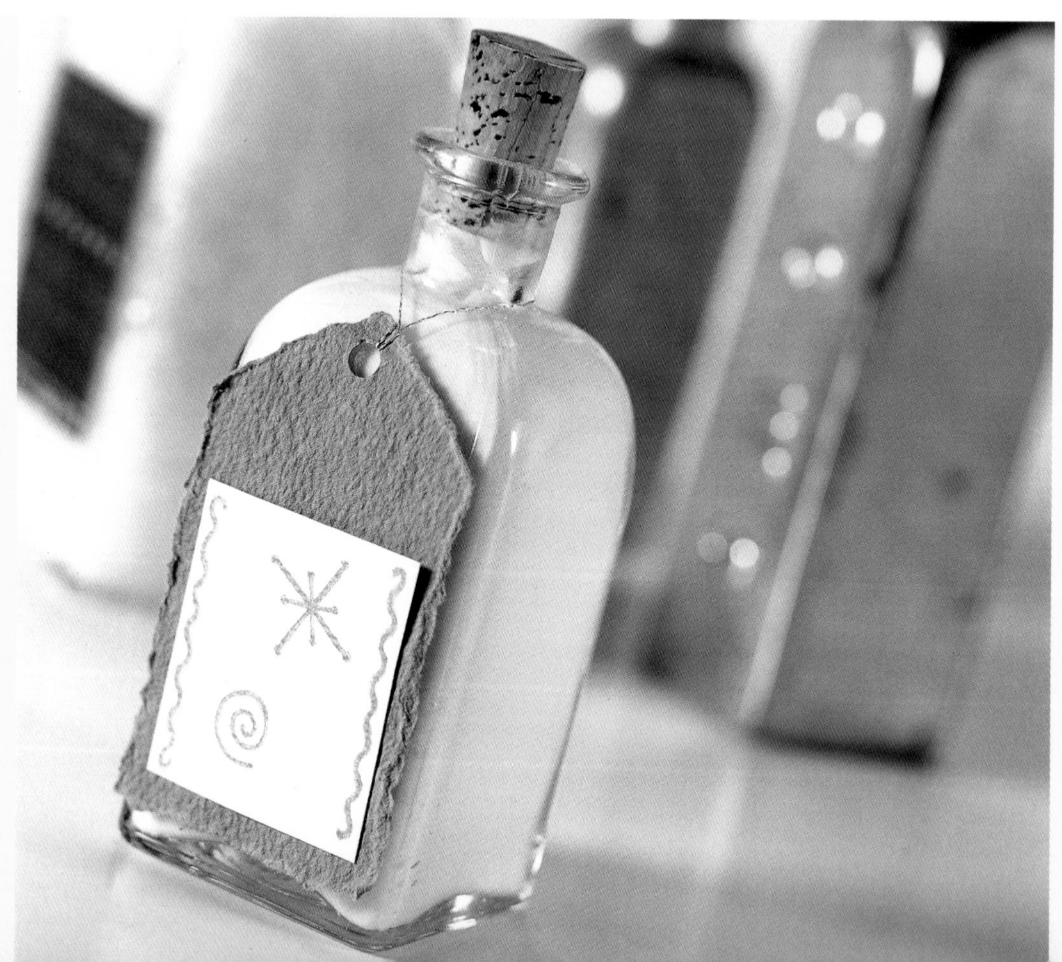

step 1 Pour the baby lotion into the bowl, add the recommended selection and quantity of essential oils, and mix thoroughly.

step 2 Insert a funnel into the mouth of the bottle and spoon in the fragranced lotion mixture. Fill the bottle and replace the stopper or cap.

step 3 Make a label by tearing blue rag paper into a gift tag shape. Cut a square of white card and glue this onto the label. Make a hole in the label and attach the gold embroidery thread. Use a gold pen to decorate the label and to write the purpose and contents of lotion, and when it was made. Tie the label around the neck of the bottle.

one

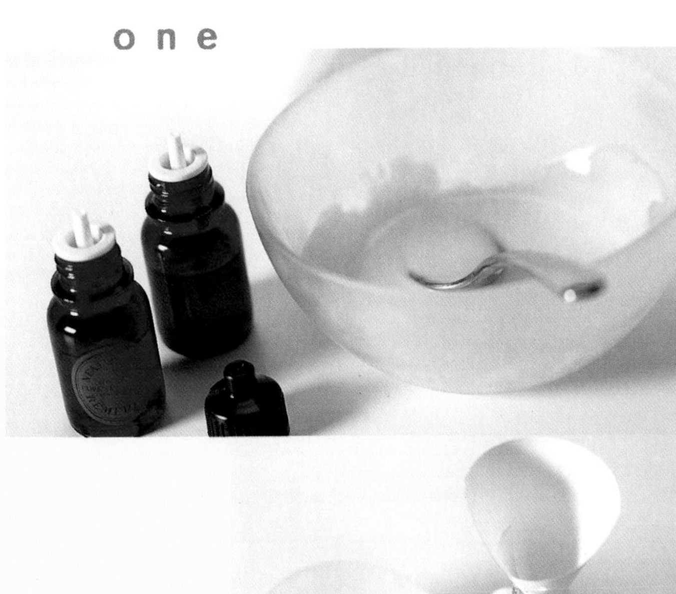

three

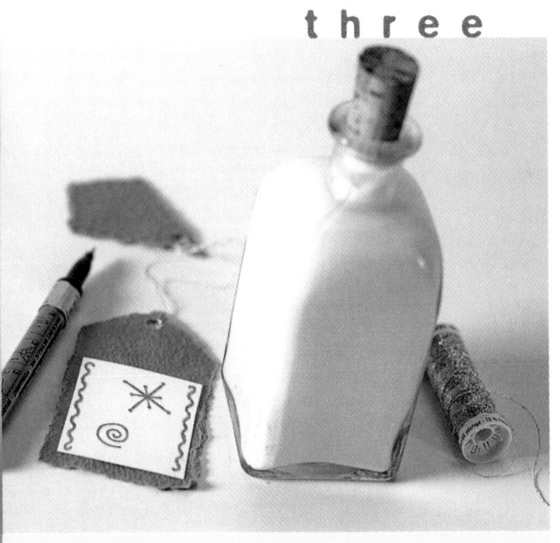

two

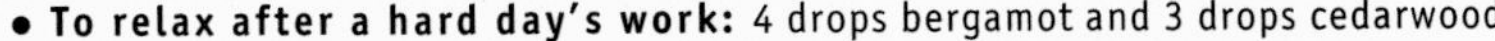

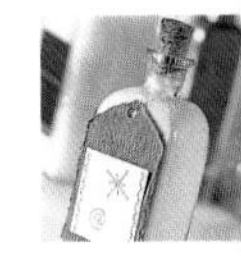

you will need

1¼ cups unscented and uncolored baby lotion

mixing bowl

spoon

selection of essential oils

small funnel

bottle with stopper or cap

blue rag paper

white card

gold thread

gold pen

- **To relax after a hard day's work:** 4 drops bergamot and 3 drops cedarwood
- **To restore energy and balance:** 3 drops cypress and 5 drops geranium
- **To stimulate and uplift the mind and spirit:** 3 drops lemon and 4 drops neroli
- **To maintain self-confidence and to aid meditation:** 3 drops rose and 4 drops sandalwood

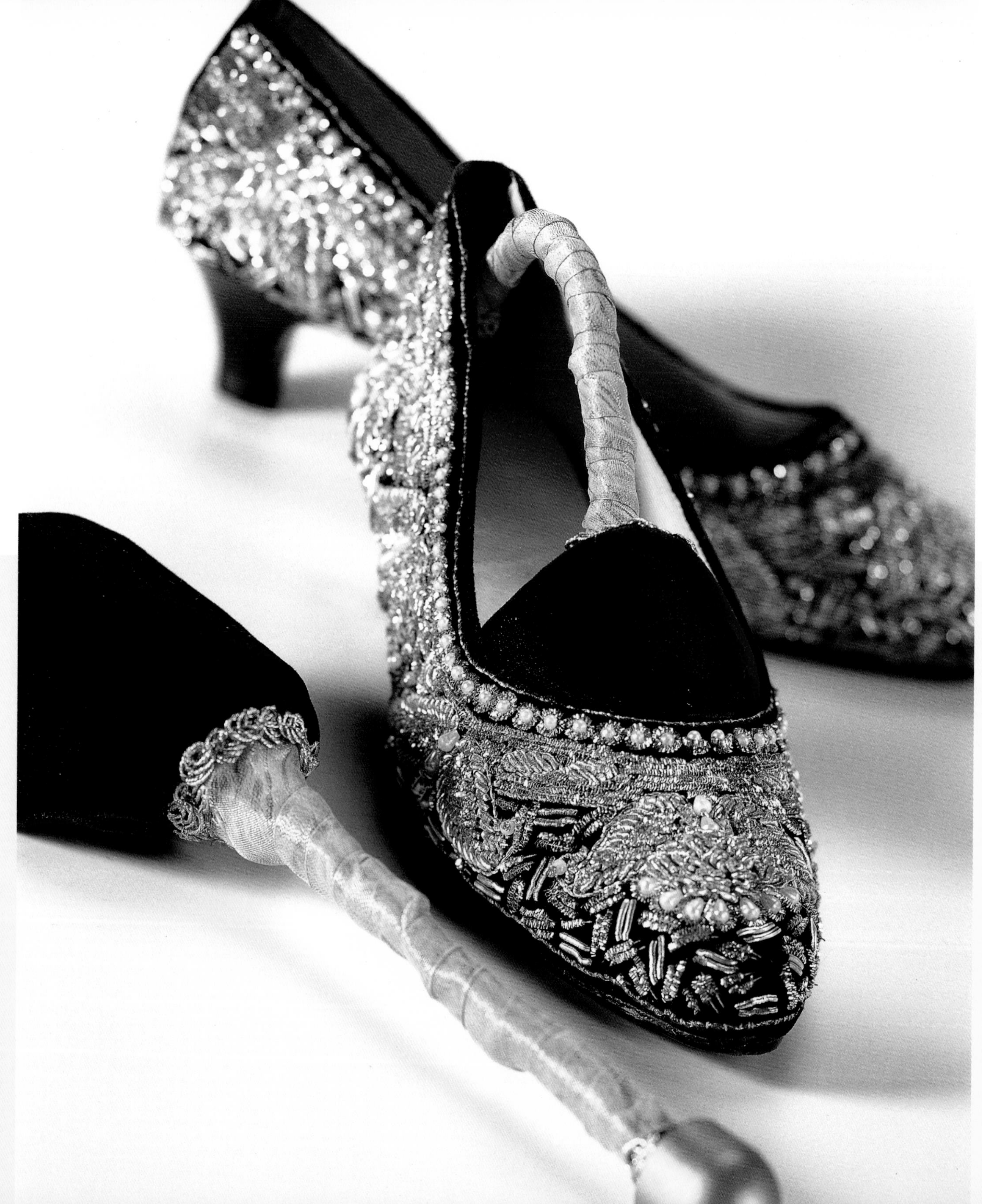

LAVENDER-SCENTED SHOE TREES

These are an indulgent must-have that will keep your favorite pair of shoes in good shape but also treat them to a light, lavender fragrancing.

To turn a pair of totally utilitarian shoe trees into something fantastic, all you need are velvet and braid trim.

one two

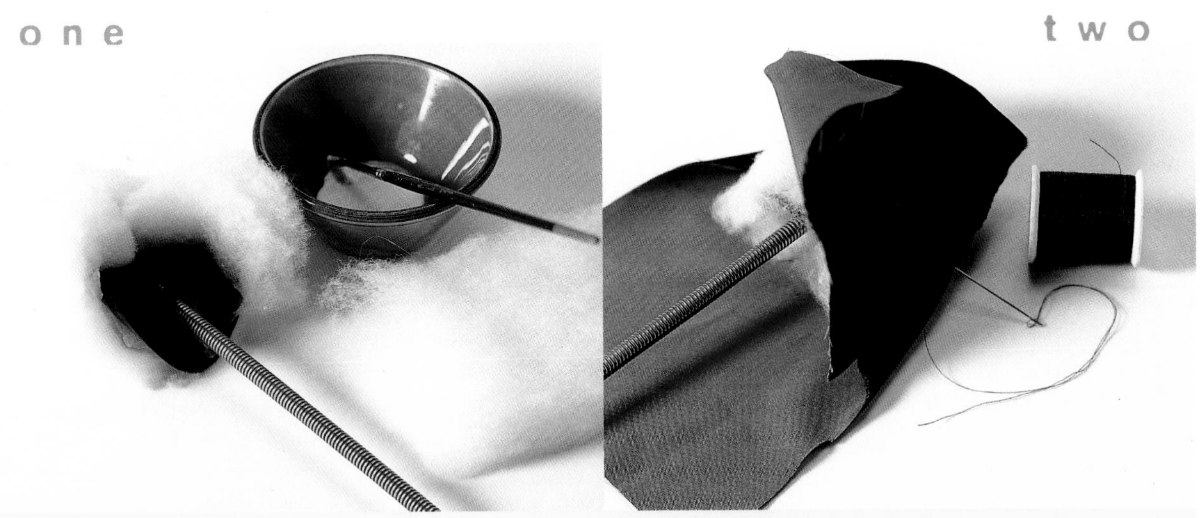

you will need

pair of plastic shoe trees

polyester batting (wadding)

scissors

fabric glue

¼ yd dark green velvet

sewing needle

dark green and gold sewing thread

dried lavender heads

gold ribbon

gold braid

gold paint and brush

step 1 Wrap batting around the toe of each tree, and cut it to fit neatly. Spread fabric glue over the toe area to secure the batting into place. Trim any excess batting.

step 2 Fit the velvet over the batting and a little way up the stem and cut it generously to fit. Position the shoe tree on the velvet and fold the fabric around the toe, tuck in the raw edges, and pin into place. Hand-sew the sides together, pulling the velvet taut as you do. Leave a large opening at the top. Repeat for the other shoe tree.

three

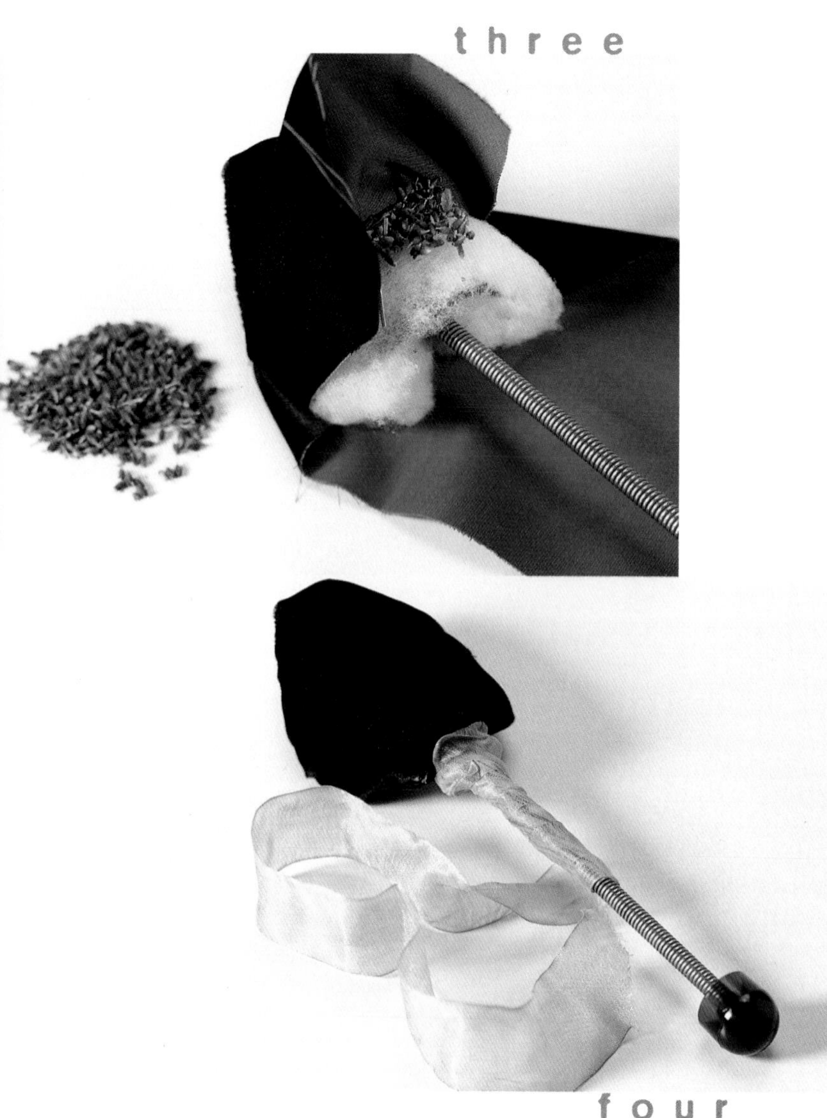

four

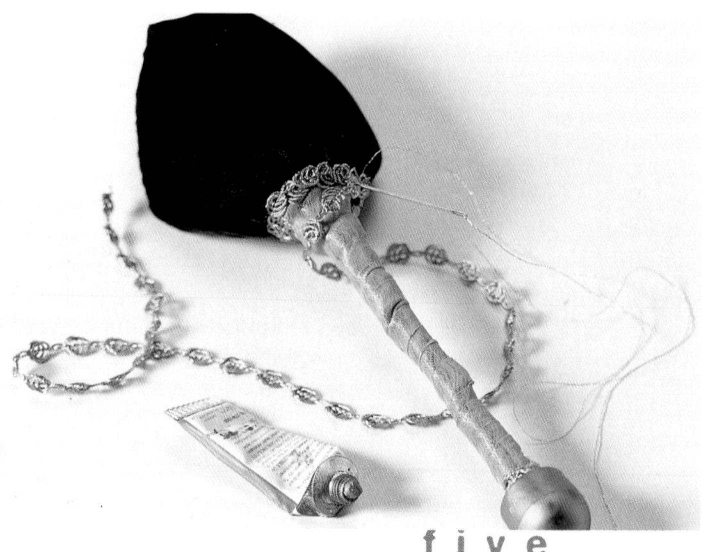

five

step 3 Stuff a handful of dried lavender heads into both openings. Pin, then hand-sew the opening, gathering and tucking the velvet as necessary. Trim any excess or bulky fabric as you work.

step 4 With fabric glue, secure gold ribbon to the stem where it meets the toe. Wind the ribbon tightly around the stem, working your way to the end. Fix the end of the ribbon in place with more fabric glue. Repeat for the other shoe tree.

step 5 Cover any untidy seams with gold braid. Attach it with fabric glue or with gold thread and hand-stitching. For the final bit of glamour, paint the end of the shoe tree gold.

LAVENDER HAND CREAM

Delicate lavender essential oil and rich coconut oil combine to create an ideal moisturizing cream that has a heady, sensual fragrance. By substituting the lavender oil with rose, musk, or peppermint essential oils, you can make a hand cream to suit your every mood.

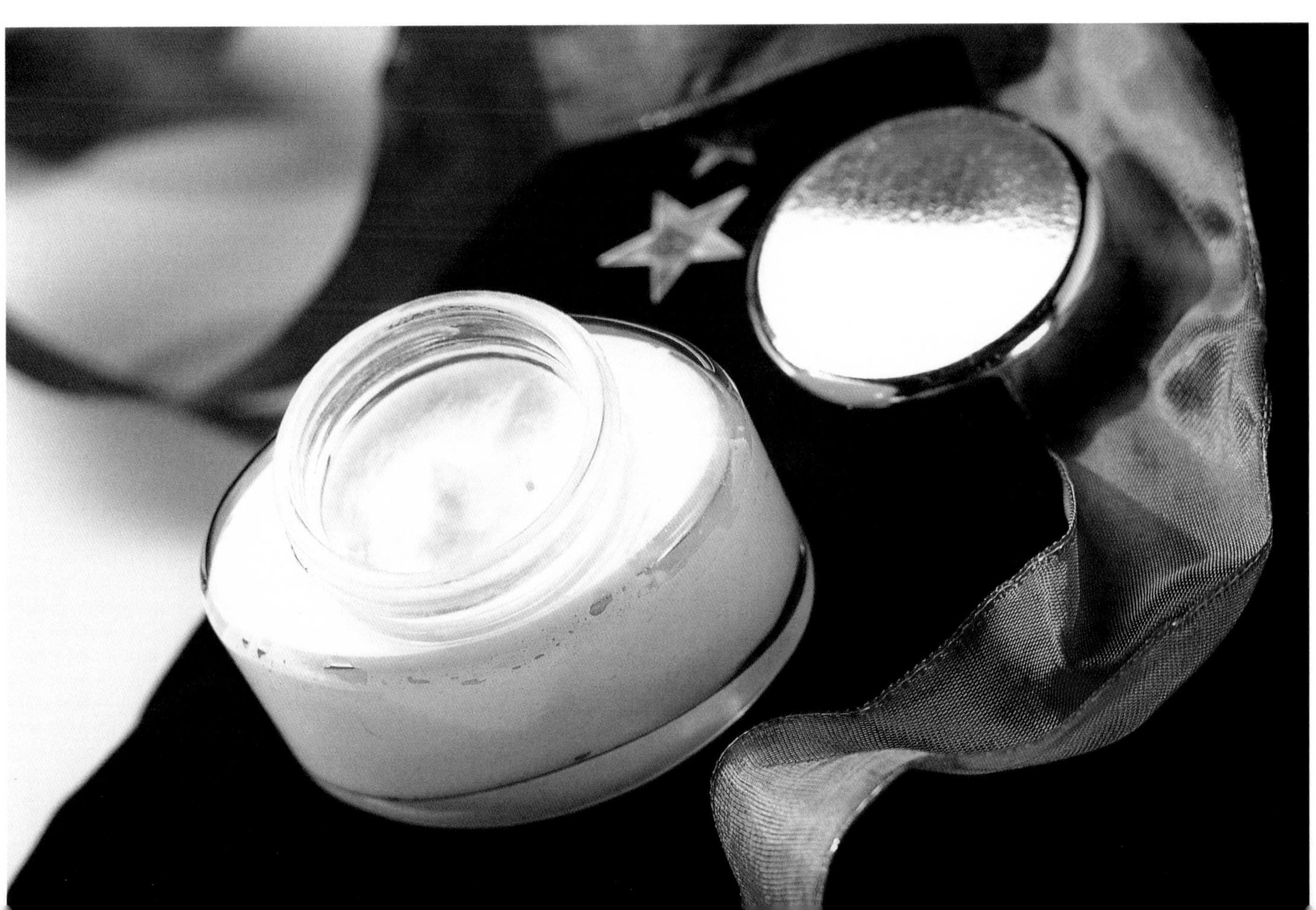

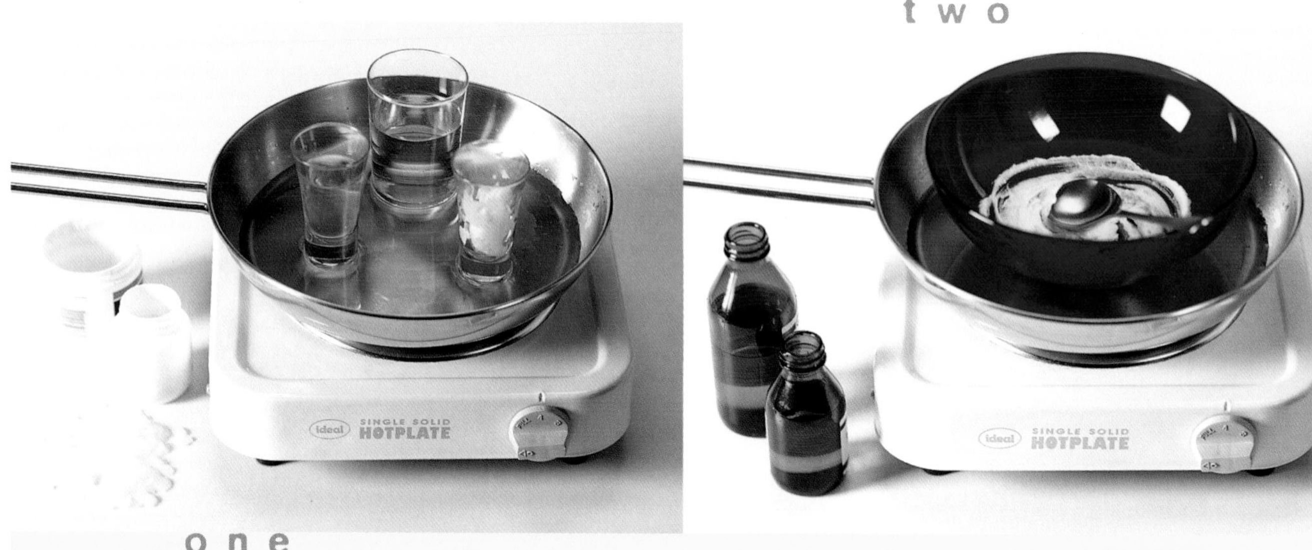

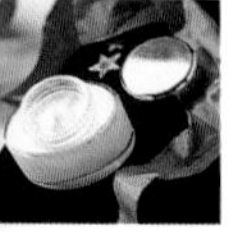

you will need

2 Tbsps white wax or beeswax

3 tsps cocoa butter

2 tsps coconut oil

3 small heatproof containers

skillet or saucepan

heatproof mixing bowl

2 Tbsps liquid paraffin

2 tsps glycerine

metal spoon

½ tsp borax

2 Tbsps boiling water

lavender essential oil

sieve

lidded glass jar

step 1 Place the wax, cocoa butter, and coconut oil into separate heatproof containers. Bring a skillet or saucepan of shallow water to a boil. Place the three containers in the skillet. Lower the heat and simmer for 5 minutes or until the ingredients melt.

step 2 Pour the melted ingredients into a heatproof mixing bowl. Sit the bowl in the simmering water, topping up the water if necessary. Add the liquid paraffin and glycerine, and stir to form a creamy mixture.

step 3 Mix the borax into the 2 tablespoons of boiling water and stir to dissolve. Add this to the creamy mixture and stir to combine.

step 4 Remove the mixing bowl from the heat, and beat in 3 to 4 drops of lavender oil. To remove lumps, force the mixture through a sieve. If you want to strengthen the fragrance, beat in an extra 1 to 2 drops of lavender oil.

step 5 When the mixture is cool, spoon it into a glass jar and replace the lid. Label the jar, specifying which essential oil was used and when the hand cream was made.

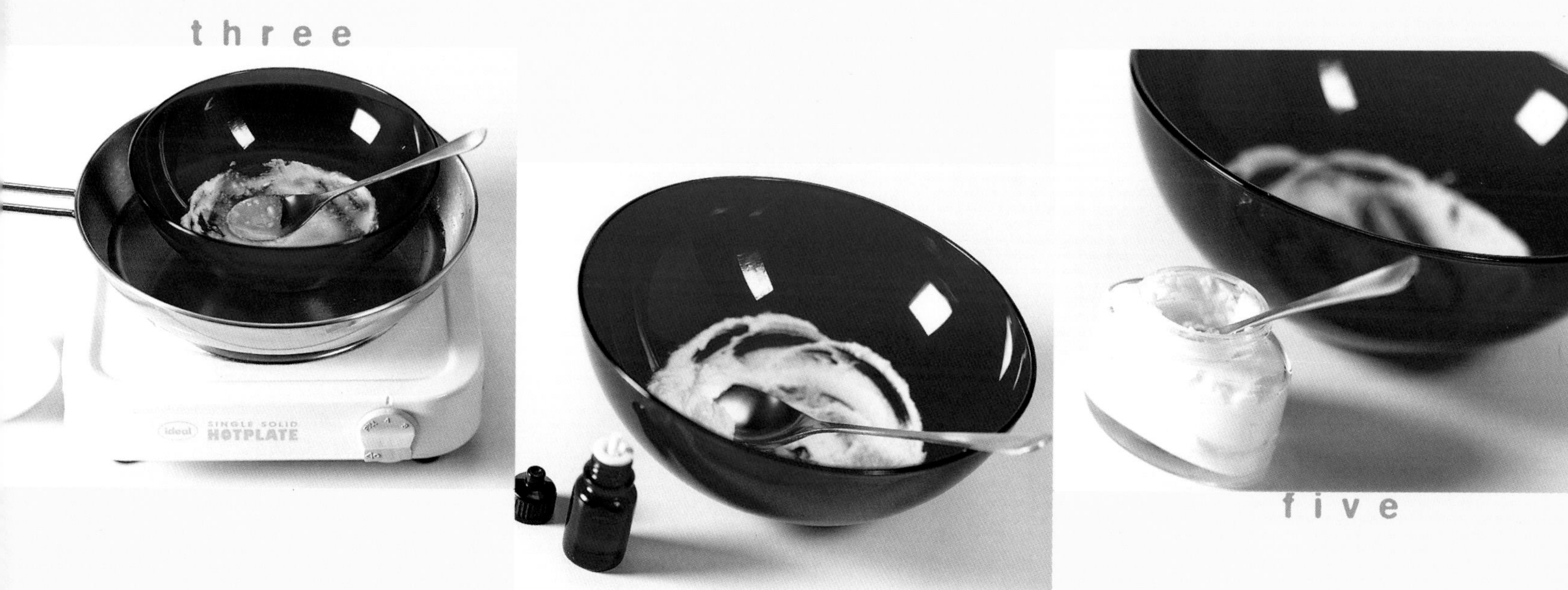

6

chapter

the aro

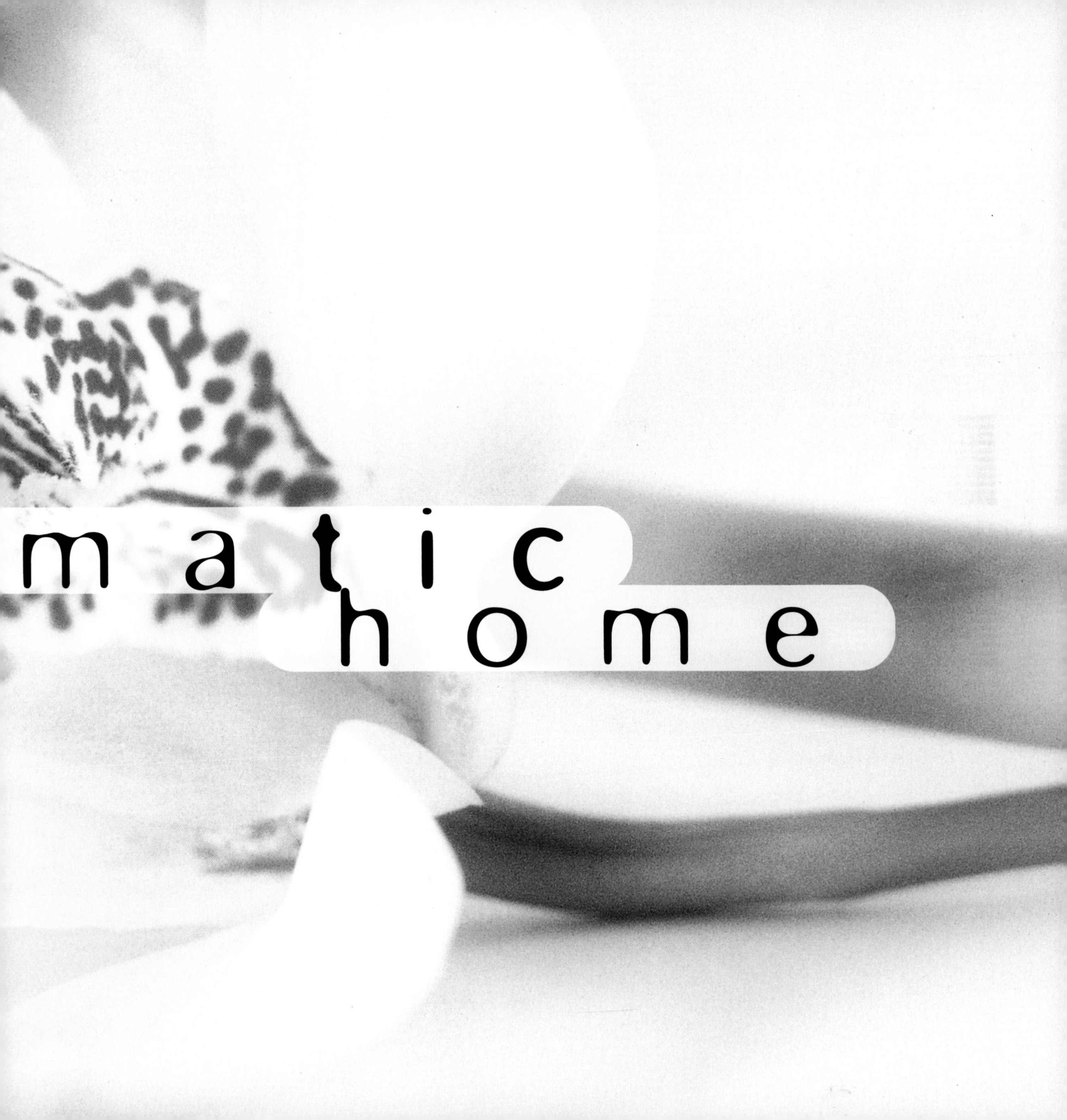

matic
home

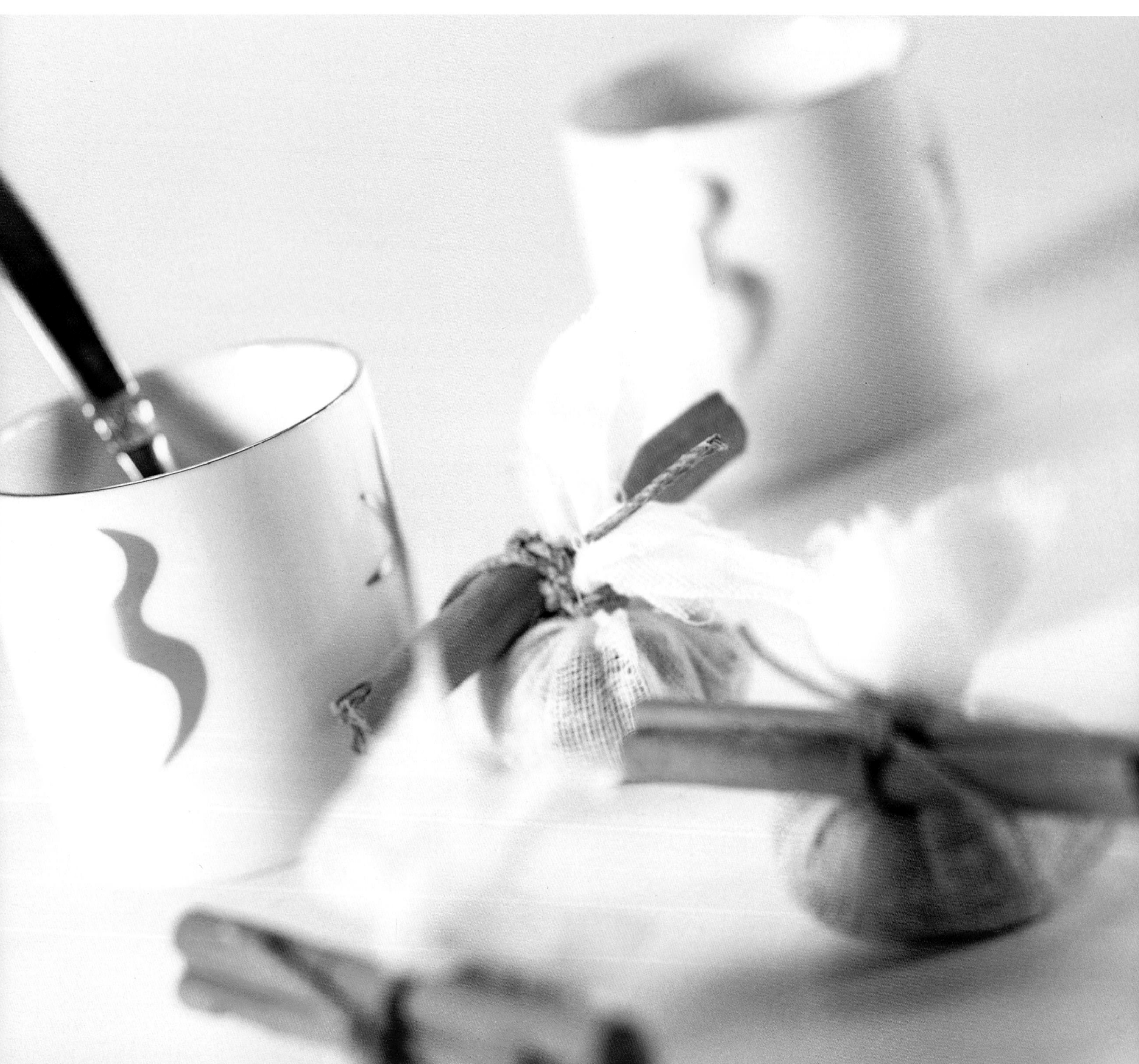

MULLED SPICE BUNDLES

To make the perfect drink for a cold winter's evening you may have to travel no further than your cupboard. Into a metal saucepan, pour a bottle of red wine and immerse the spice bundles. Heat gently for ½ to one hour and your cosy tipple is ready! This recipe will make five spice bags.

one

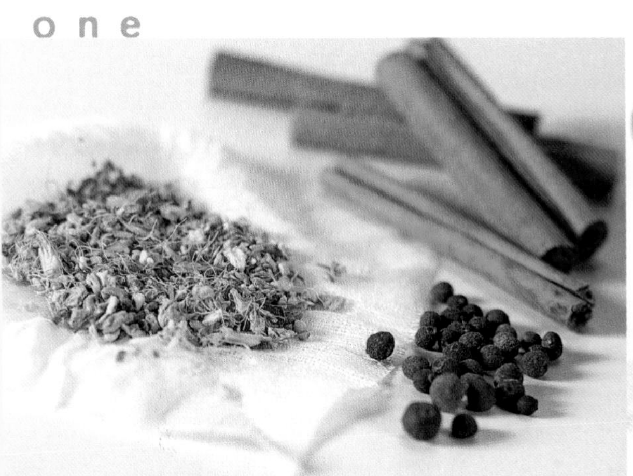

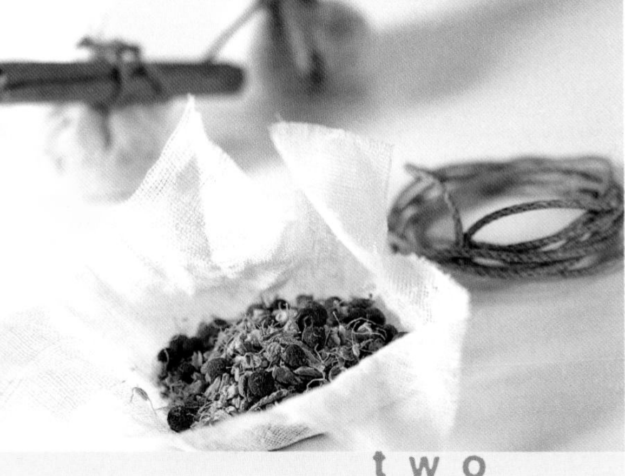

two

step 1 Cut out five 5-inch squares of cheesecloth and lay them on a smooth surface. Mix the spices, except the cinnamon, together in a small bowl. Place a teaspoon of the mixture into the center of each cheesecloth square.

step 2 Gather up the corners of each square and tie together with twine. Attach a cinnamon stick to each bundle with more twine. Trim the twine to neaten.

you will need

cheesecloth (unbleached butter muslin)

scissors

chinese five spice powder

1 tsp whole peppercorns

1 tsp ground cloves

1 tsp ground fennel

1 tsp ground ginger

½ tsp ground caraway seeds

small bowl

natural twine

small cinnamon sticks

CLOVE AND CINNAMON CANDLES

Plain beeswax candles have a lovely natural fragrance, but you can add spicy notes to its fragrance with cinnamon and clove. Remove the ribbon before lighting the candle and never leave a lit candle unattended.

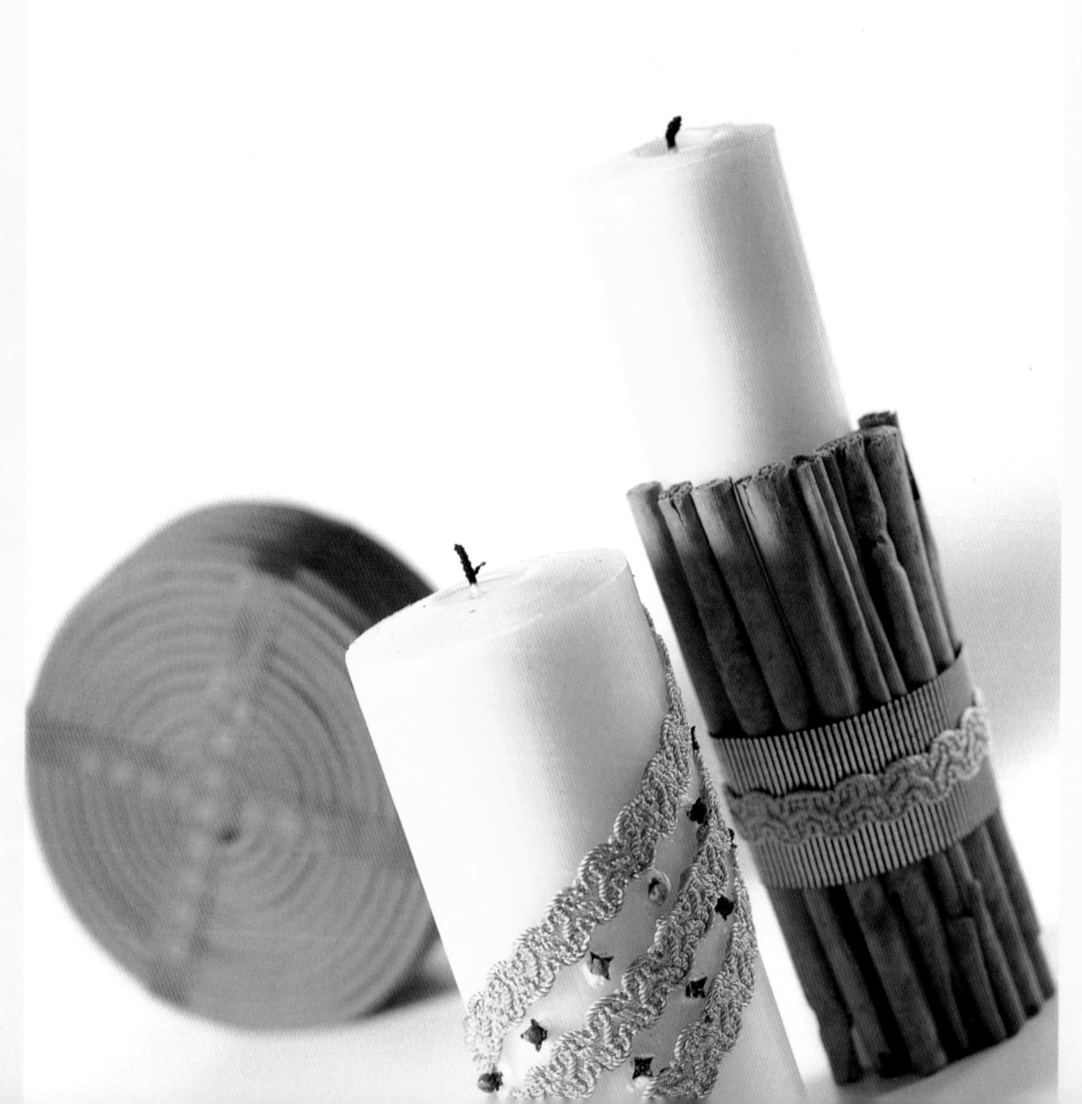

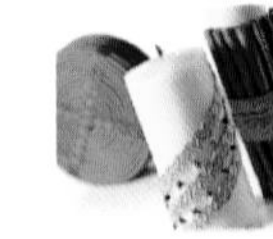

one

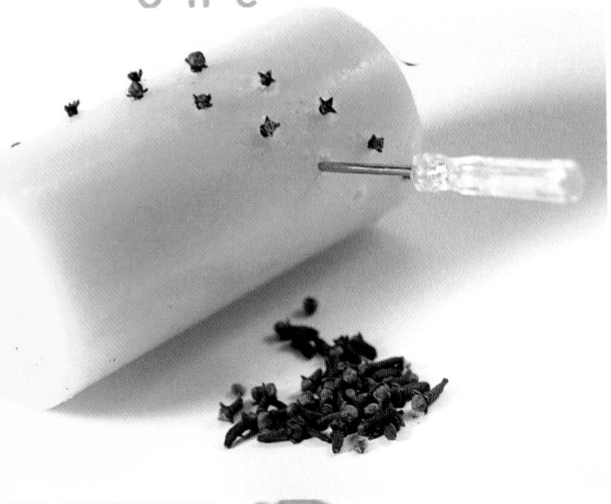

two

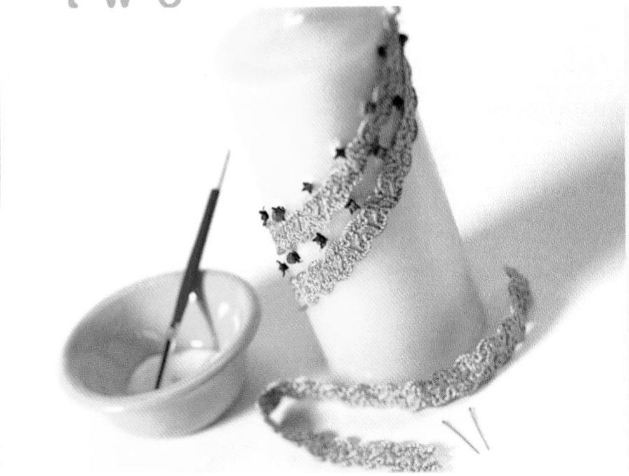

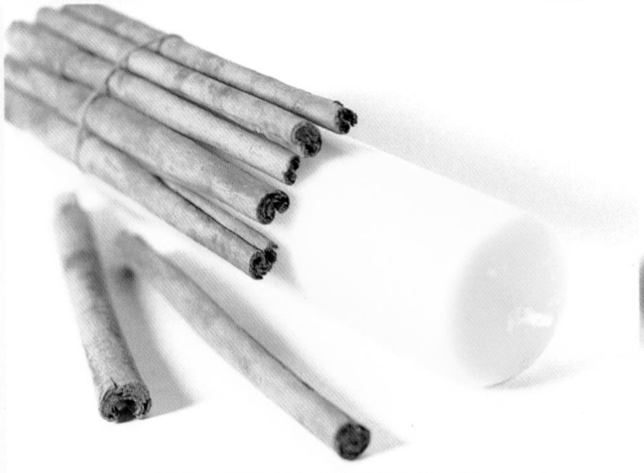

one

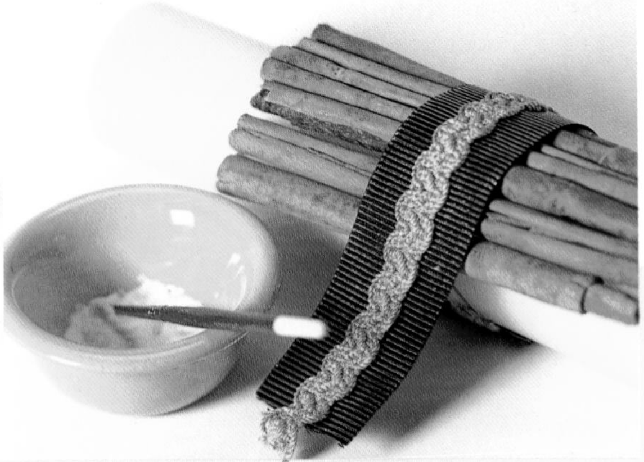

two

you will need:

beeswax candles

pencil

bradawl

pocket lighter

whole cloves

gold braid or ribbon

fabric glue

dressmaking pins

rubber band

cinnamon sticks

ribbon

clove candle

step 1 Use a pencil lightly to mark where you want the cloves to be studded into the candle. Heat the tip of the bradawl with a lighter and carefully pierce the candle at the marked spots. Place the cloves into the holes.

step 2 Apply glue to the wrong side of the gold braid and stick it onto the candle so that the braid echoes the pattern of the cloves. Use dressmaking pins to hold the braid in place while the glue dries.

cinnamon candle

step 1 Wrap a rubber band around the candle and insert the cinnamon sticks behind it to cover half the circumference of the candle.

step 2 Place a length of ribbon around the candle so that it covers the rubber band. Secure the ribbon with glue, using pins to hold it in place while the glue dries.

ROSE-SCENTED HEART SWAG

This romantic swag looks striking and smells heavenly. It can be hung anywhere and the fragrance will last for ages due to the presence of orris root powder and gum benzoin tincture, which are both preservatives.

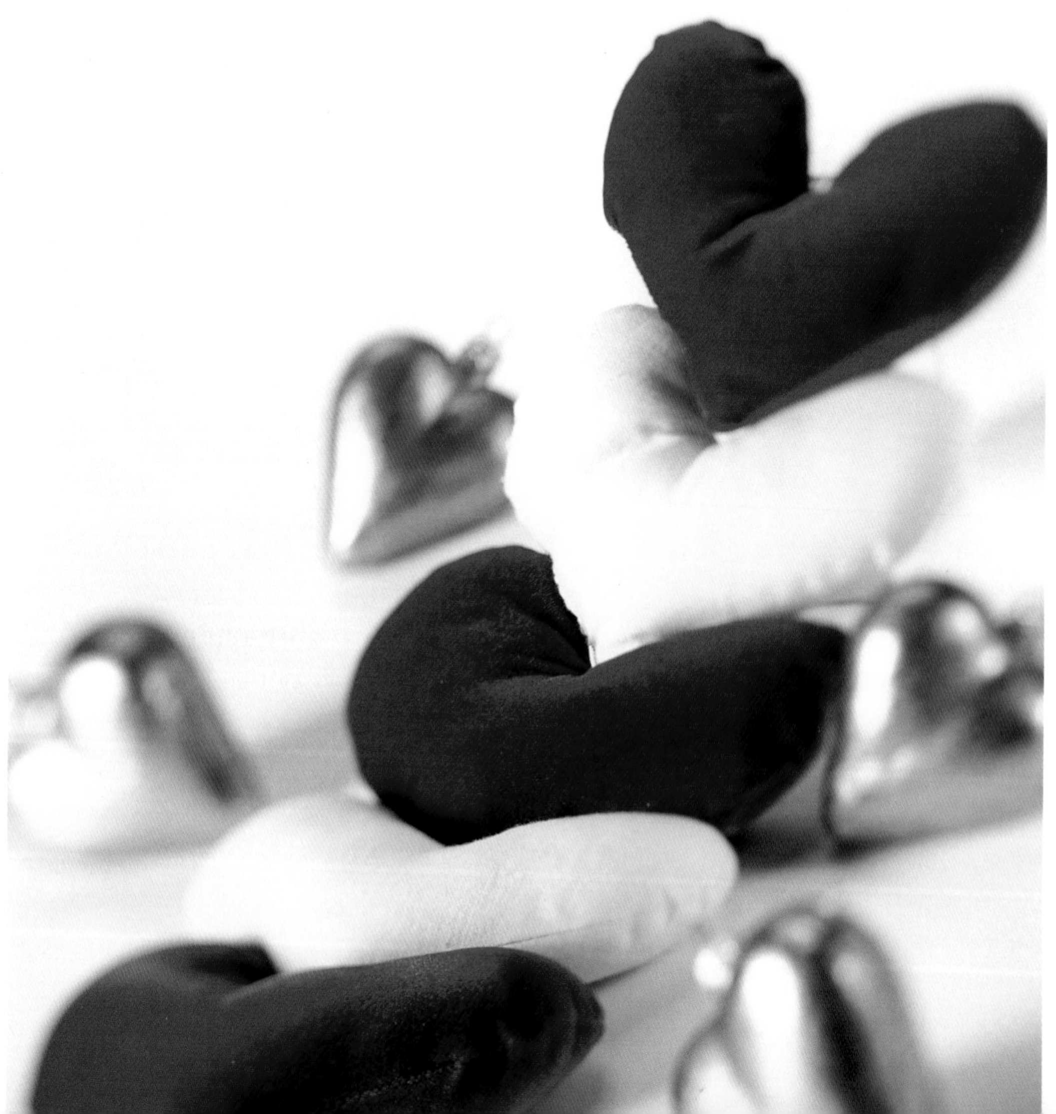

step 1 Trace and cut out the heart template on page 143. Draw around it six times on the red velvet and four times on the calico. These are sufficient to make three red hearts and two cream hearts. Cut them out carefully.

step 2 With right sides facing, machine-sew around the edge of two hearts of the same fabric. Leave an opening at the side, as shown. Turn the heart right way out, using a pencil to push out the curves and peaks. Press into shape with a warm iron. Repeat to make the remaining four hearts.

step 3 Blend together thoroughly the orris root powder, gum benzoin tincture, and rose essential oil. Spoon 2 tablespoons into each of the velvet hearts. Do not put the mixture into the calico hearts as the orris root will stain the fabric. Fill all the hearts with batting.

step 4 Close the openings with small hand stitches. Arrange the hearts in a vertical line, colors alternating, so that the peak of one heart fits neatly into the dip of the one below. Hand-stitch them together with a few well-placed stitches on the back of the swag. To hang, attach a loop of gold thread to the top of the first heart.

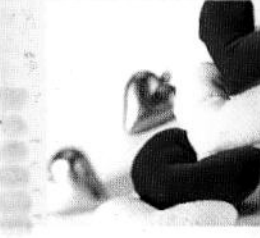

you will need:

red velvet

unbleached calico

pencil

scissors

sewing machine

sewing needle

red and cream sewing thread

iron

6 Tbsp orris root powder

10 drops gum benzoin tincture

10 drops rose essential oil

small mixing bowl

tablespoon

polyester batting (wadding)

gold thread

one

two

three

four

PINK PETAL CHRISTMAS DECORATIONS

Instead of buying Christmas decorations, it's even easier to make them. These decorations look wonderful hung on the tree for Yuletide or used in place of traditional potpourri and displayed in a decorative container.

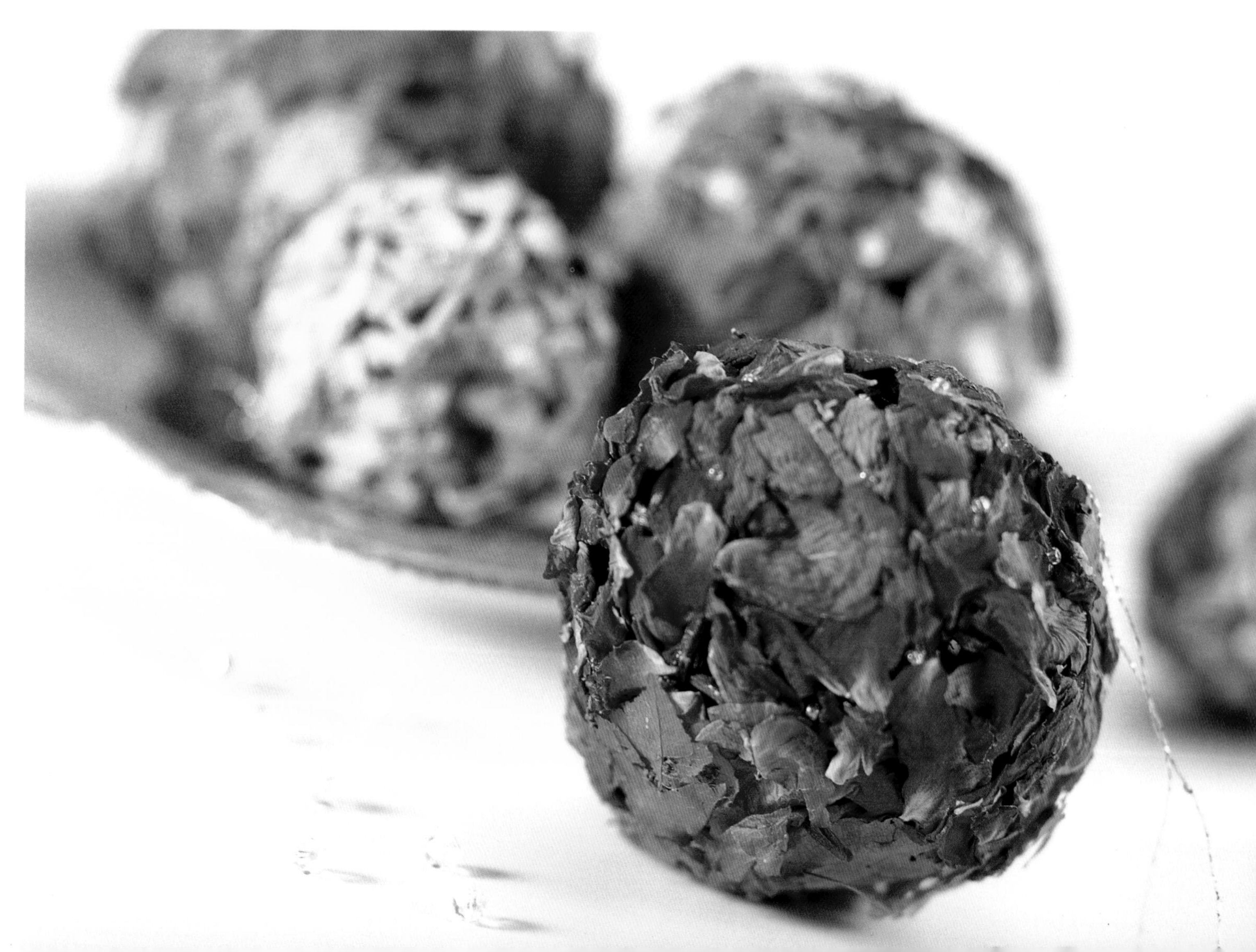

one

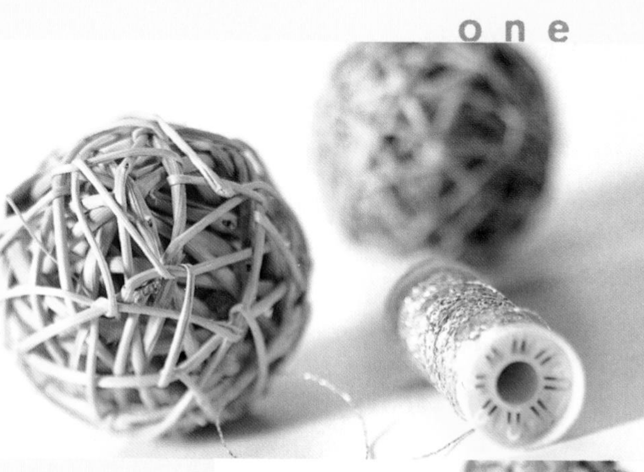

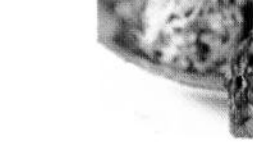

you will need:

small twig sphere

gold thread

scissors

white craft glue

pink and red rose potpourri petals

small, clear glass beads

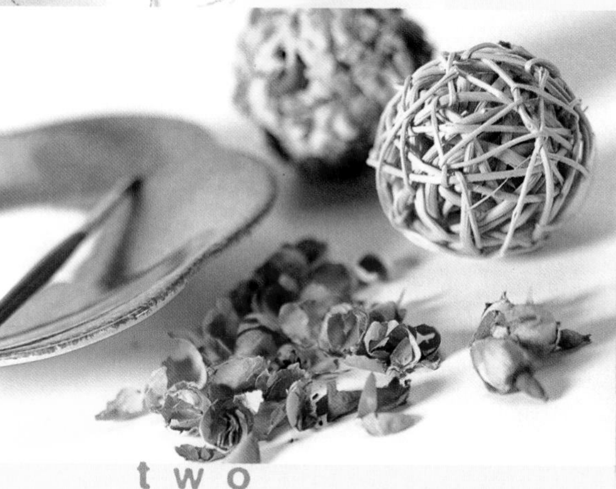

two

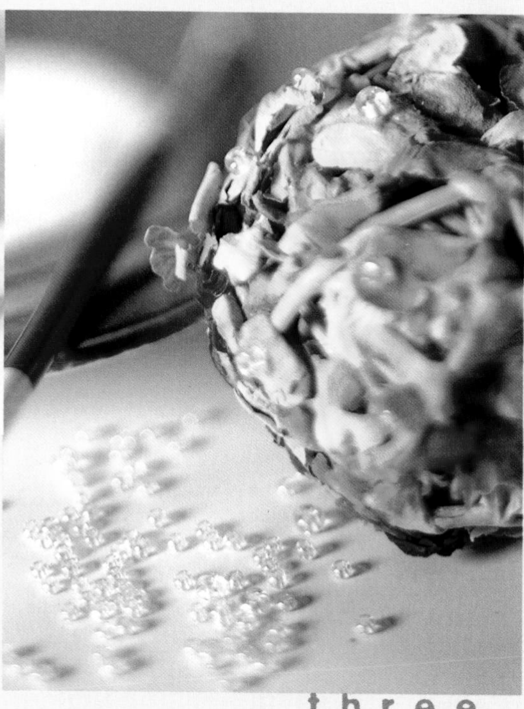

three

step 1 Thread a short length of gold thread through a section of the twig sphere and tie it to create a loop.

step 2 Brush glue all over the sphere. Press the petals into the glue and cover the sphere completely.

step 3 To finish, glue clear glass beads in a random pattern onto the sphere. These beads will sparkle when they catch the light.

MANDARIN-SCENTED TWIG BUNDLE

This festive decoration is ideal for hanging on the front door. Its mandarin scent will welcome guests to your home. Mandarin essential oil is said to have warming and soothing properties.

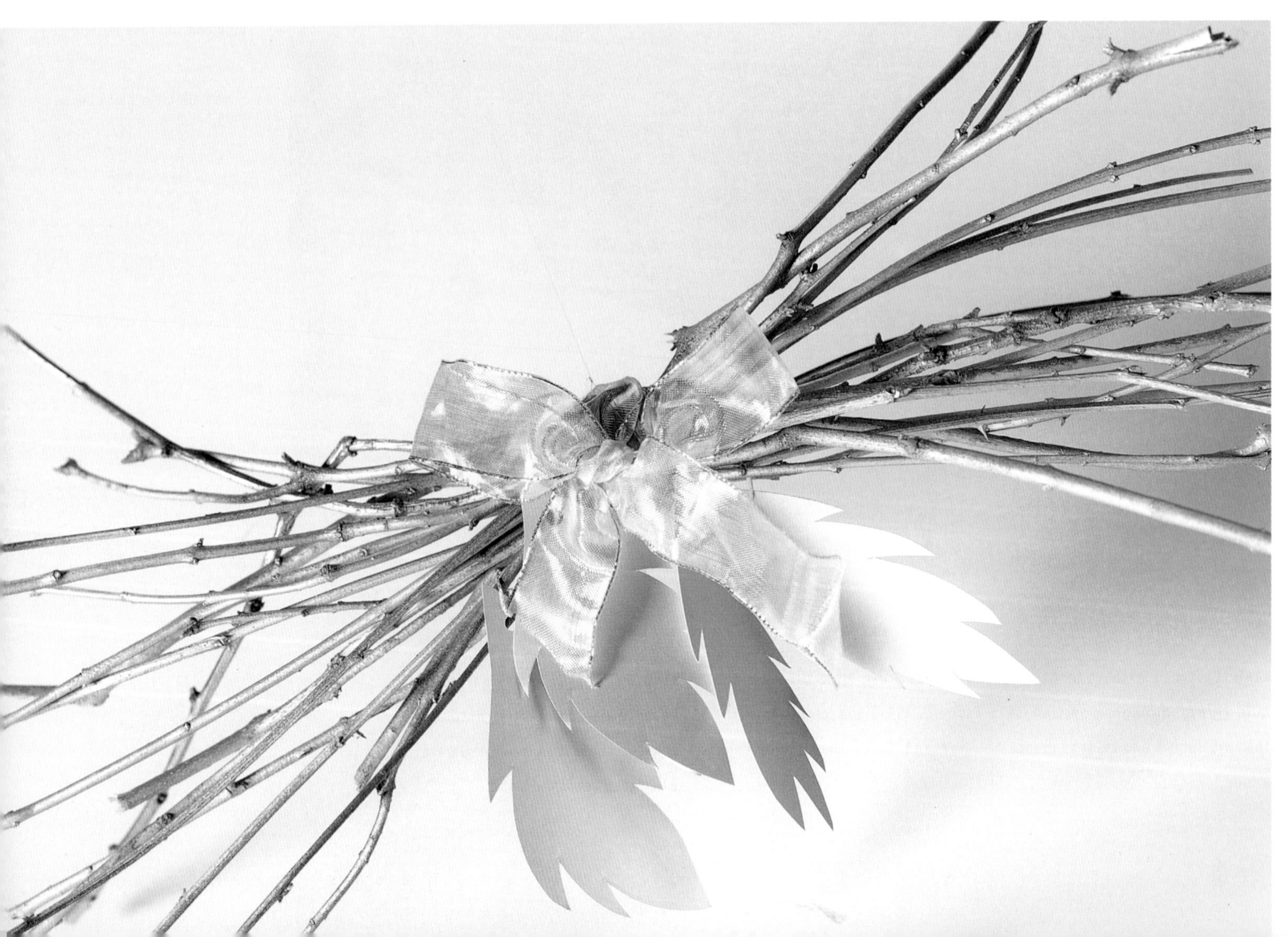

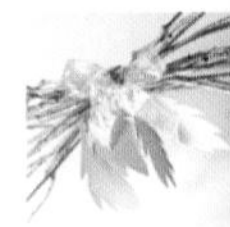

you will need:

selection of twigs about 24 to 30 inches in length

silver spray paint

silver card

pencil

scissors

mandarin essential oil

hole punch

twine

silver thread

iridescent ribbon

nylon fishing line

step 1 Lay the twigs on a piece of newspaper in a well-ventilated area and spray them silver. Do one side first and allow to dry, then turn the twigs over to spray the other side. Leave to dry.

step 2 Trace and cut out the leaf-shape template on page 142. Draw around them onto the back of the silver card and cut them out. Apply 2 to 3 drops of mandarin essential oil to the back of each leaf. Make a hole in the stem-end of each leaf with a hole punch.

step 3 Form the twigs into a bundle and find the midpoint. Bind them together at this point with twine. Pass silver thread through the hole in each leaf and attach them to the center of the bundle. Tie a decorative ribbon around the bundle to hide the twine. To hang it, attach a loop or a length of nylon fishing line.

one

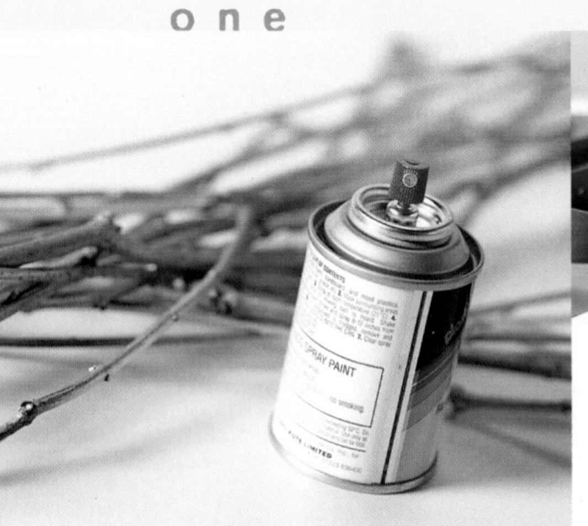

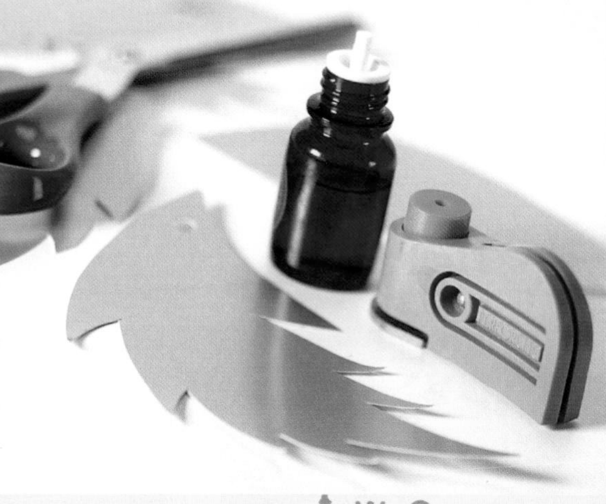

two

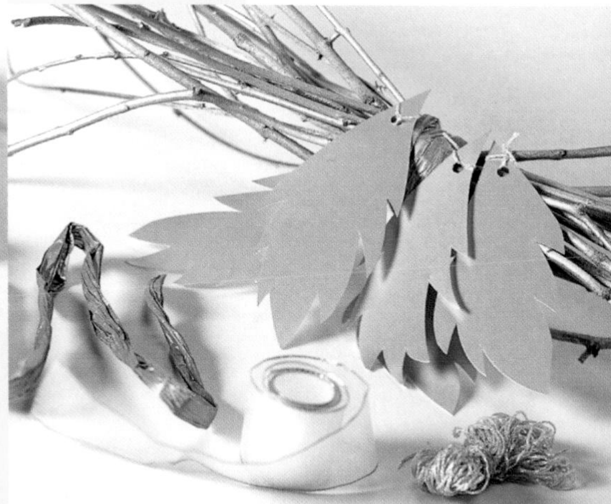

three

CELESTIAL ESSENTIAL OIL BURNER

Give an ordinary essential oil burner some extra sparkle by decorating it with silver stars and swirls. When the night light is burning, the glass star sequins will catch the light to give a celestial glow.

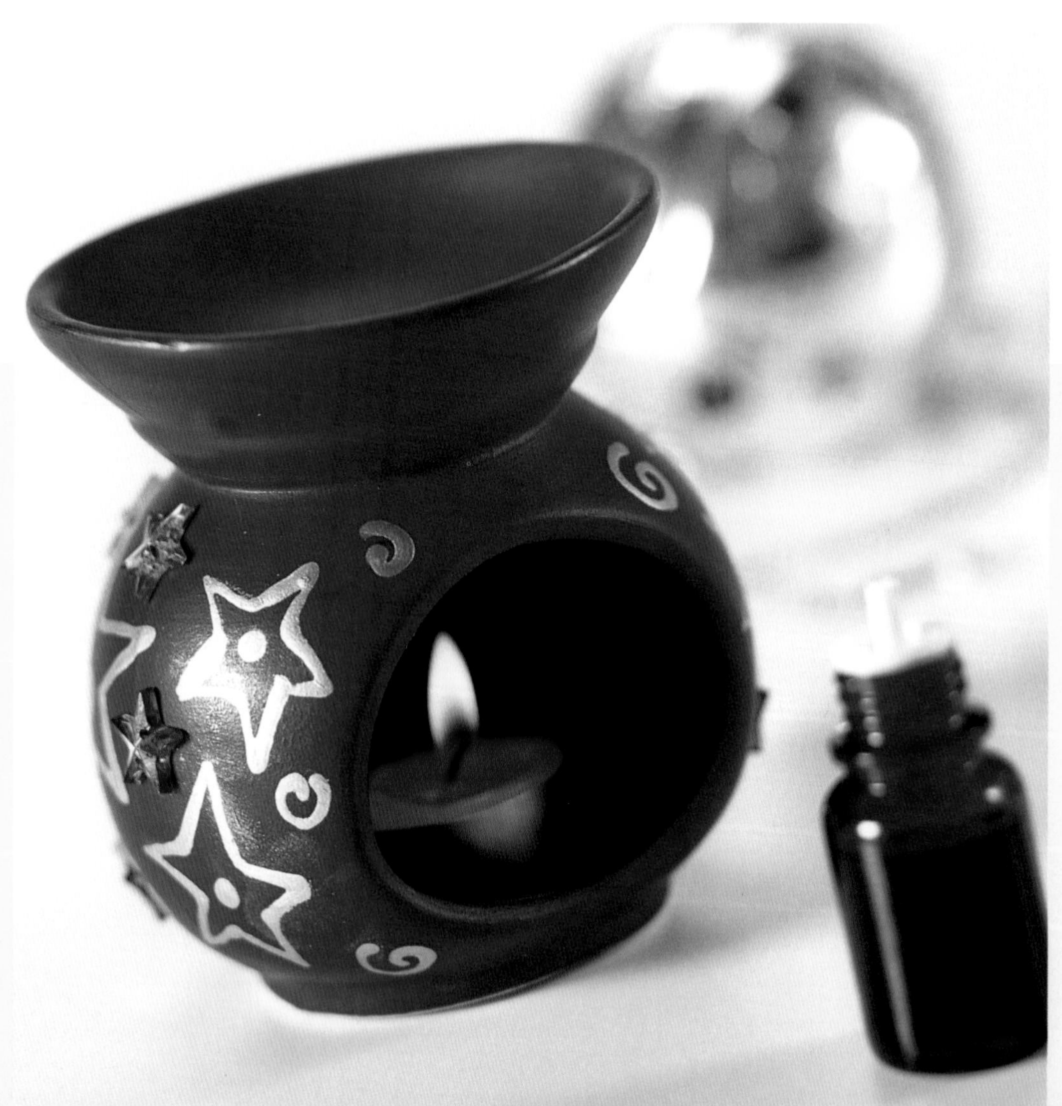

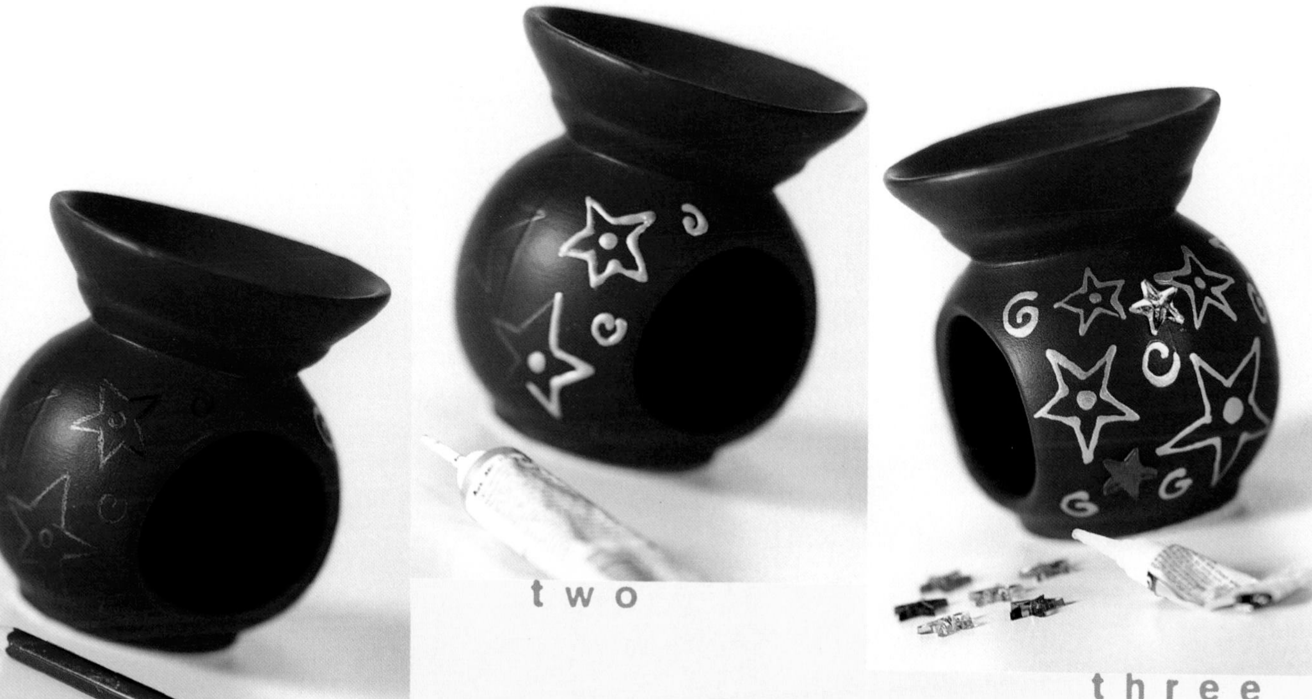

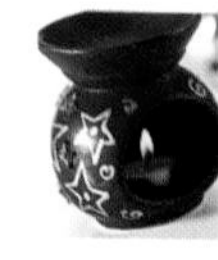

you will need:

dark blue clay essential oil burner

pencil

eraser

tube of silver ceramic paint

red glass star sequins

strong, heat-resistant glue

step 1 Work out the design you would like to paint onto the burner or use the pattern guide on page 139. Using a faint pencil, draw the pattern onto the burner. Remove any mistakes with an eraser.

step 2 Test the tube of silver ceramic paint on a piece of paper before you start work on the burner. When you are happy with the flow of paint, simply go over your pencil lines. Take care not to smudge the paint.

step 3 When the paint is dry, use a very strong and heat-resistant glue to stick the glass star sequins onto the burner. Dot the sequins about so that they complement your design.

ROSEBUD TOPIARY TREE

This beautiful tree looks like it is the work of a professional, but it is in fact very easy to make, requiring patience rather than skill. In place of rosebuds you can use potpourri petals, dried leaves, and moss.

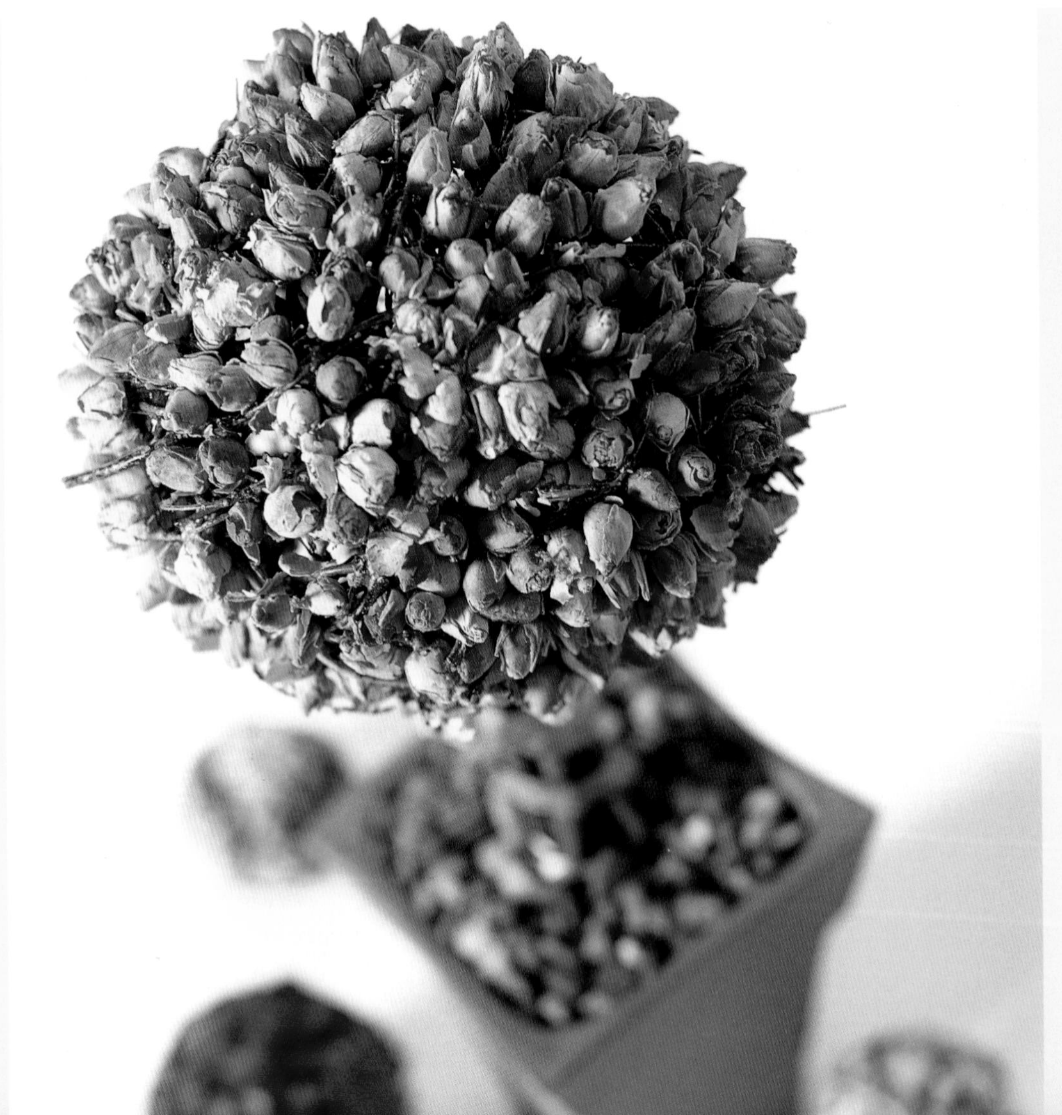

step 1 Apply a generous layer of glue onto the wicker sphere and then proceed to stick the rosebuds all over it, leaving only a small space into which the trunk can be inserted. This task is quite time-consuming and requires patience. If the glue dries, apply more.

step 2 Trim the twigs to the same length. Bundle them together and bind them tightly with gold paper twine. This is the trunk of the topiary tree.

step 3 Position the trunk into the space on the sphere. Hold it in place with florists' wire wrapped around the twigs and catching onto the exposed parts on the sphere. To further secure the trunk, apply glue to the area where the trunk and sphere touch.

step 4 Fill any gaps on the tree by gluing on more rosebuds. Cut a piece of florists' foam to fit snugly inside the plant pot. Put the shaped foam into the plant pot and push the trunk firmly into it. To finish, cover the foam with a handful of gravel.

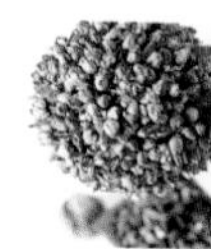

one

two

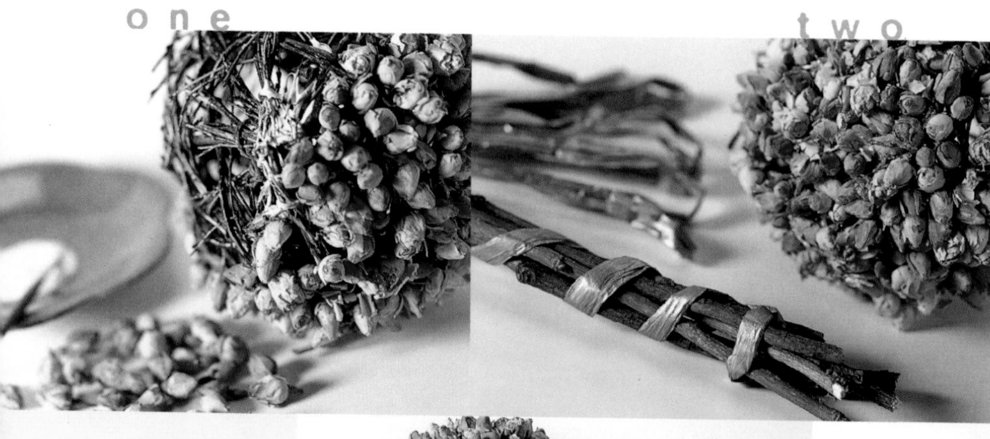

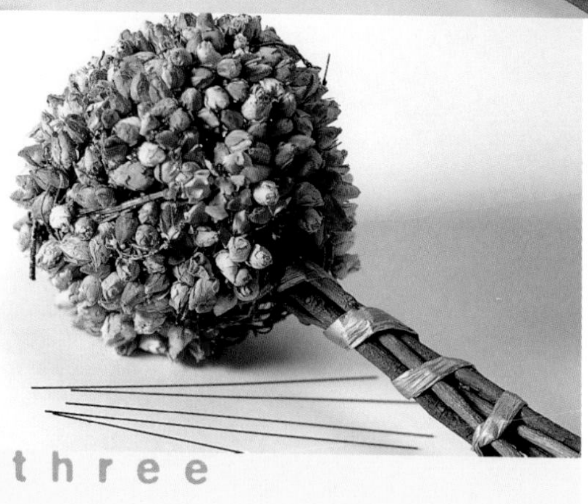

three

four

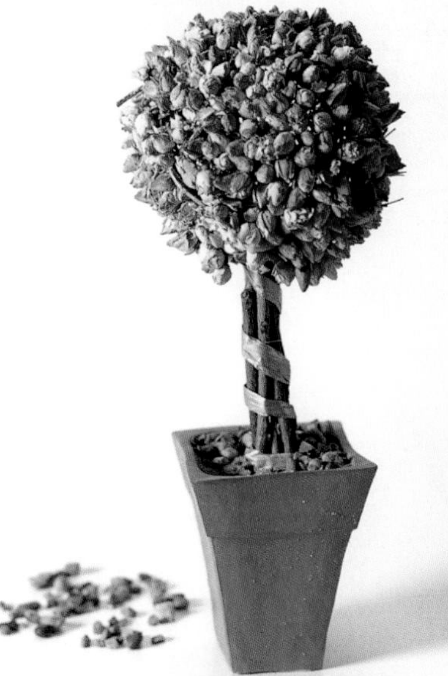

you will need:

wicker sphere

white craft glue or woodworking glue

dried pink rosebuds

4—5 straight twigs of similar thickness

garden cutters

gold paper twine

florists' wire

terracotta plant pot

block of florists' foam

gravel

LAVENDER FAN

This very feminine fan can decorate a wall and fill a room with scent. It is an interesting alternative to potpourri or scented room spray.

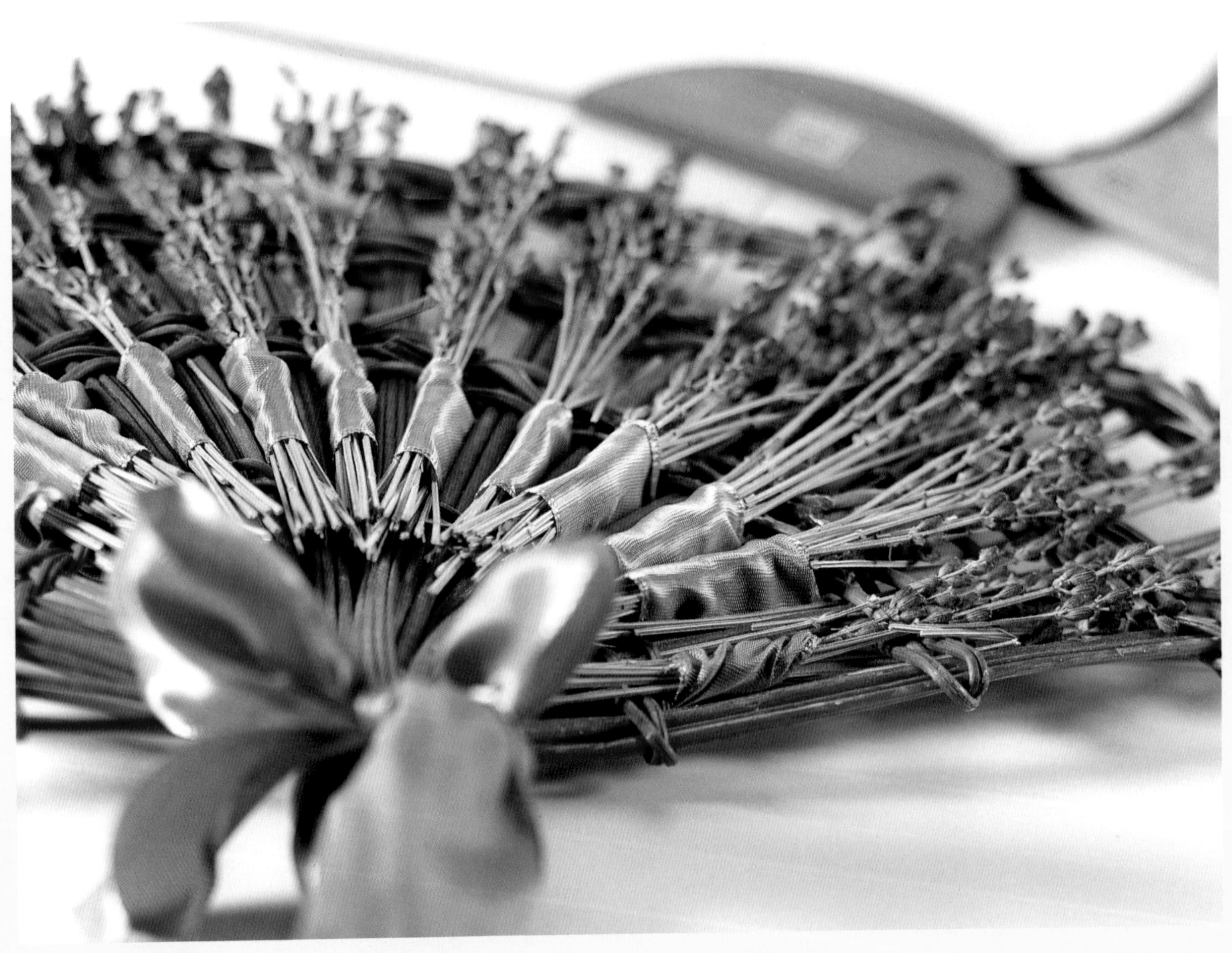

step 1 Weave the lavender sprigs in and out of the wickerwork so that the flower heads frame the outer edge of the fan and fill the top segment.

step 2 Continue weaving, but this time fill the middle segment with flower heads. Trim any overhanging stems as you work. Spread out some lavender sprigs on top of the wickerwork, as shown. Arrange these sprigs in small bundles and fix them in position with glue.

step 3 When the glue is dry, weave a length of ribbon in and out of the wickerwork and the lavender sprigs in the lowest segment. The ribbon will conceal uneven stems and also help keep the lavender in place.

step 4 Wind another length of ribbon around the handle and finish with a bow.

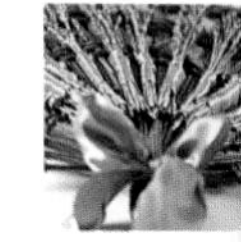

you will need:

wicker fan

dried lavender sprigs

scissors

white craft glue

wired purple ribbon

one

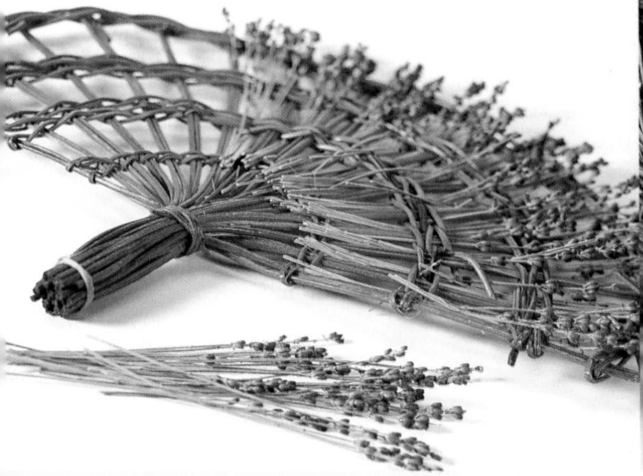

two

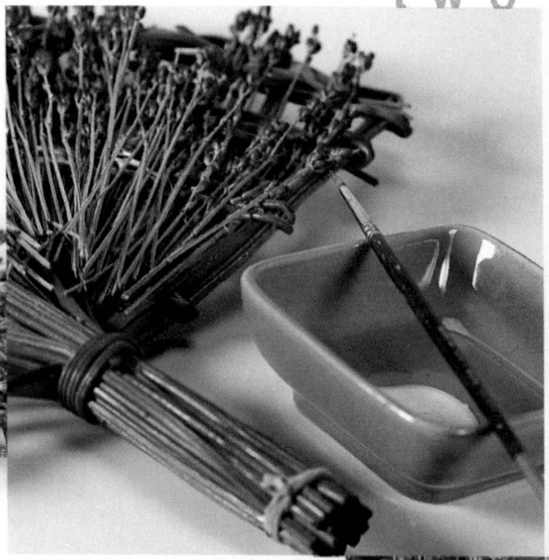

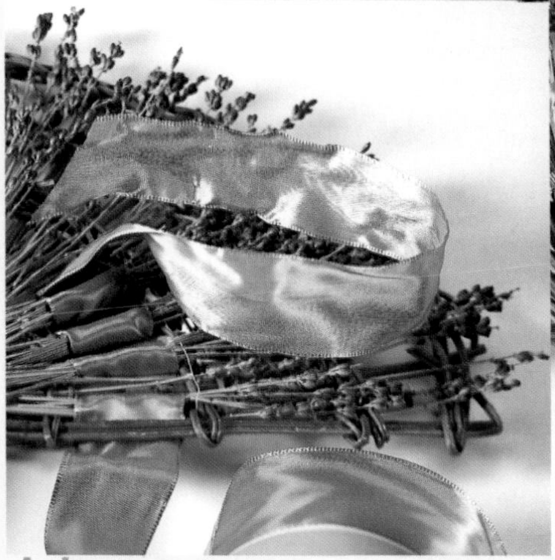

three

four

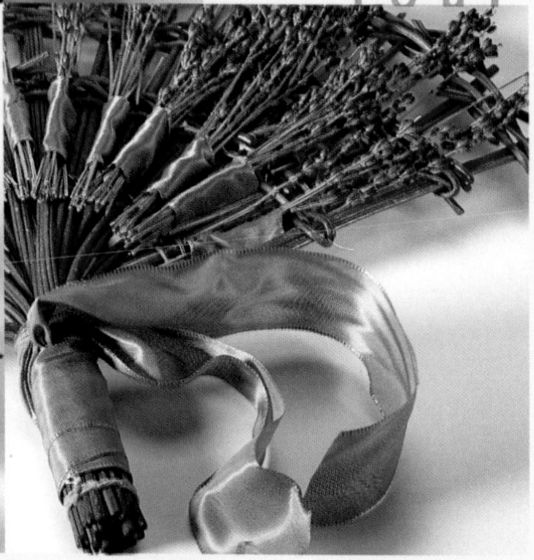

PADDED AND SCENTED COAT HANGERS

Treat your clothes well and they will last for years. Heavy coats and jackets that hang on inadequate hangers throughout the year can look tired when you bring them out. These beautiful yet functional hangers will solve this problem.

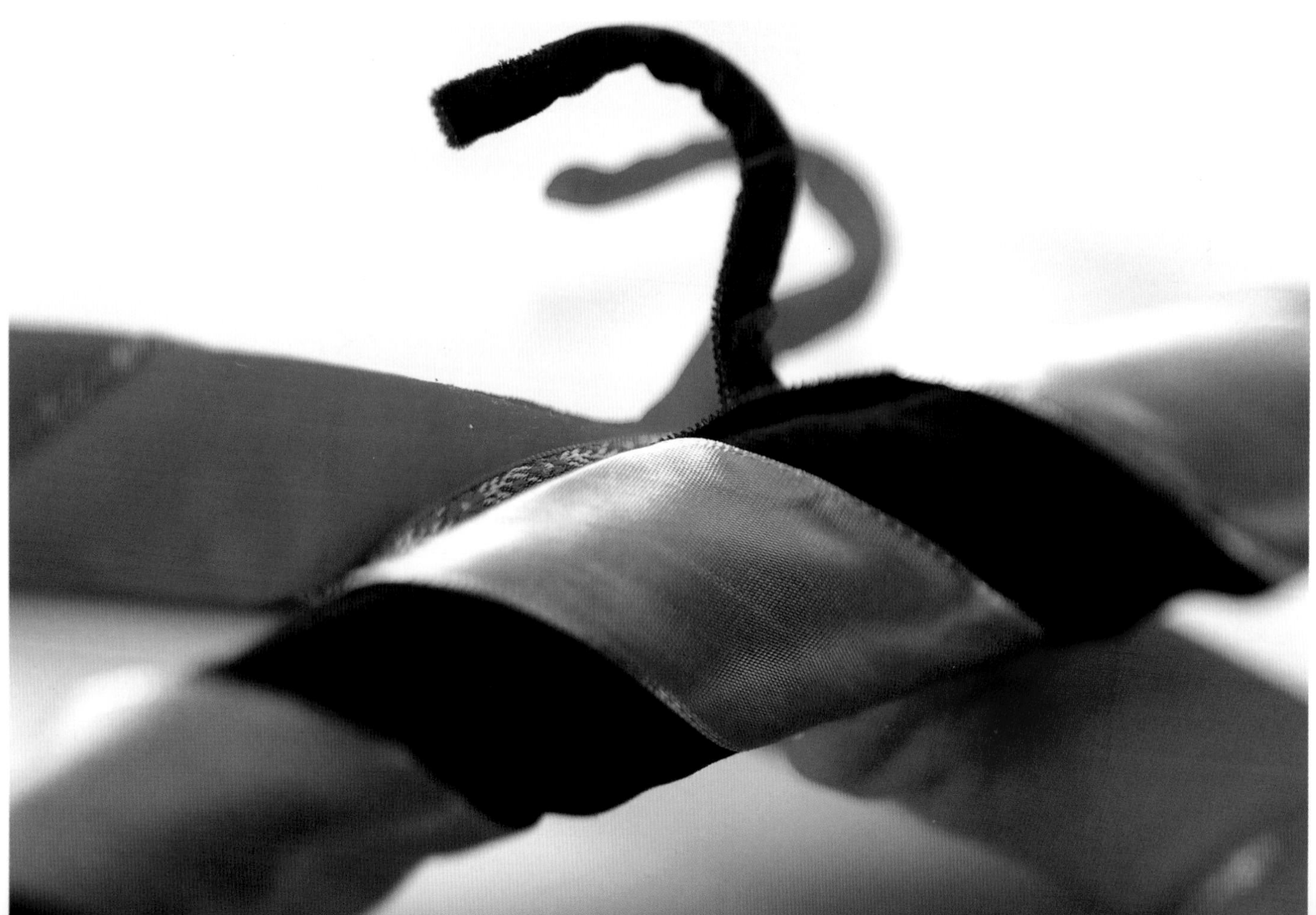

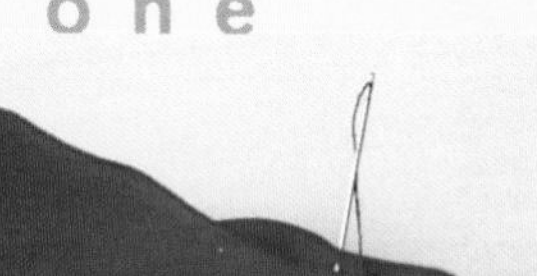

one

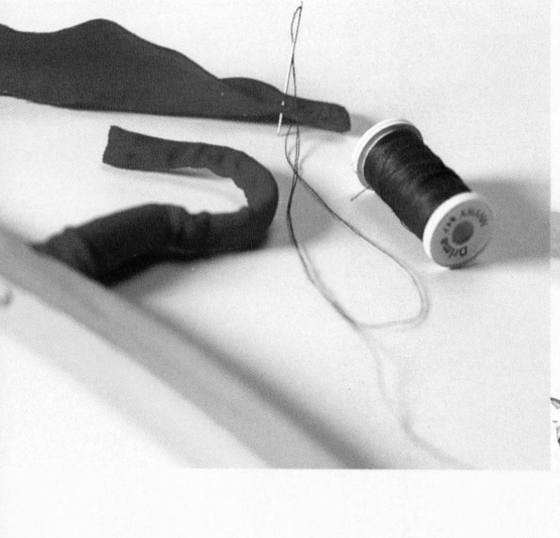

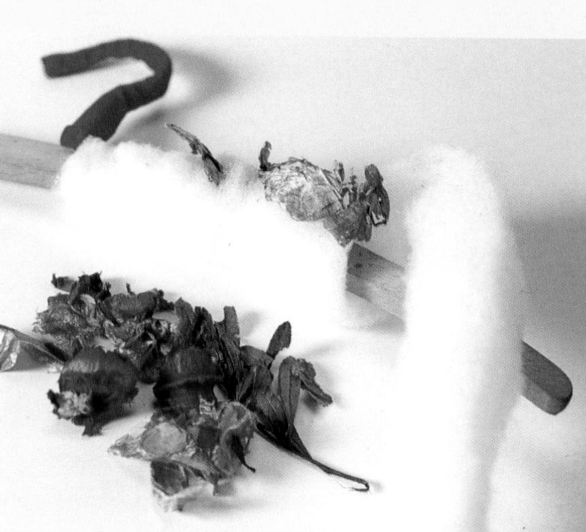

two

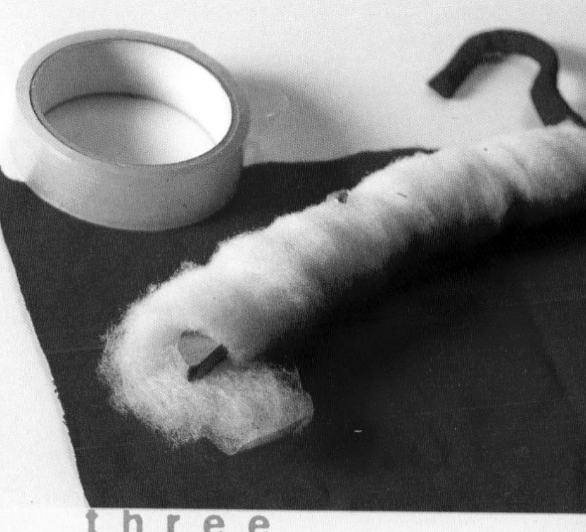

three

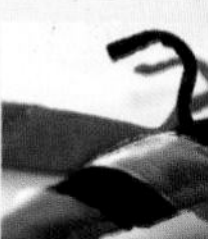

step 1 Cut a strip of velvet that is slightly longer than the hanger hook. Fold the strip in half lengthways, wrong sides facing, and then turn over the raw edges using pins to secure. Hand-stitch the edges together and close one end to make a narrow tube. Slide it over the hook to cover it.

step 2 Cut two strips of batting, both at least the same length as the hanger. Use tape to fasten the end of one strip of batting to the hanger near the hook. Wind it around the hanger, placing potpourri petals under the batting as you work toward the end of the hanger. At the end, fix the batting with more tape.

step 3 Complete the other end of the hanger as in step 2. Lay out the velvet and place the hanger on it. Cut the velvet to fit, making sure that it is wide enough to cover the hanger and making a small allowance for a seam.

you will need:

wooden coat hanger

red velvet

pair of scissors

sewing needle

red sewing thread

polyester batting (wadding)

tape

potpourri of your choice

dressmaking pins

ribbon

four

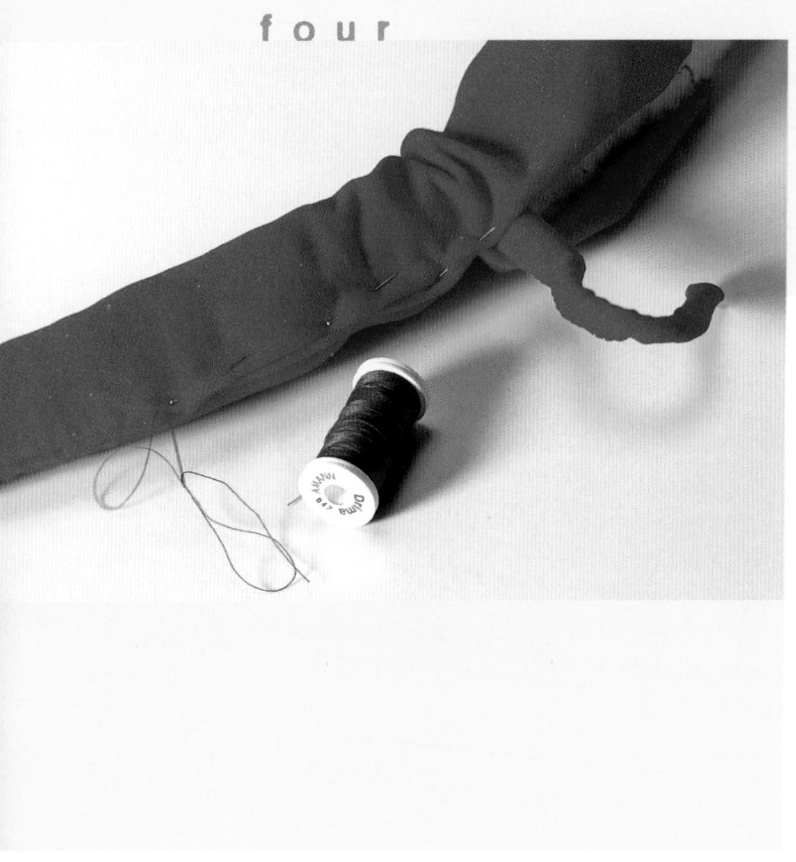

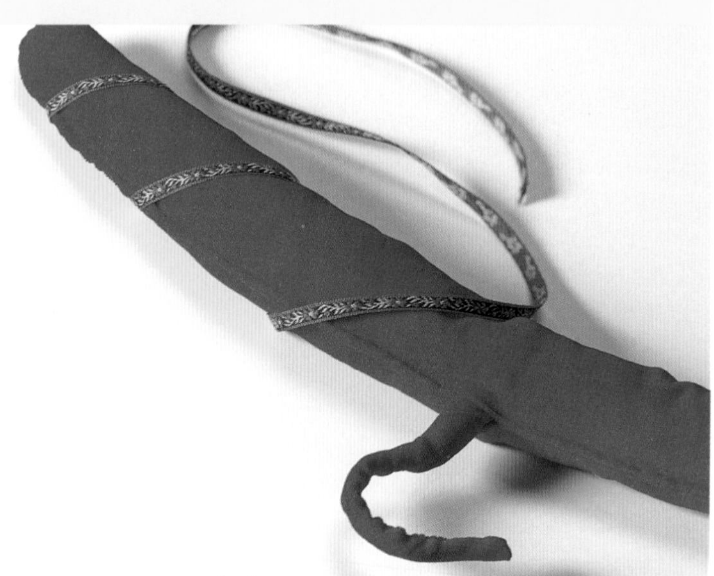

five

step 4 Fold the velvet over the hanger so that the raw edges are at the top. Pin the velvet tightly, folding in the raw edges as you pin. Hand-stitch the seam using tiny running stitches and pulling the velvet taut as you work.

step 5 Secure the velvet cover on the hook to the hanger cover with a few stitches. Wind ribbon around the hanger, securing each end with a couple of stitches.

GINGHAM SOAP BAGS

Soaps are popular gifts and you can make such a gift extra-special with this sweet soap bag. The bag can be used later to hold potpourri or other bathing accessories.

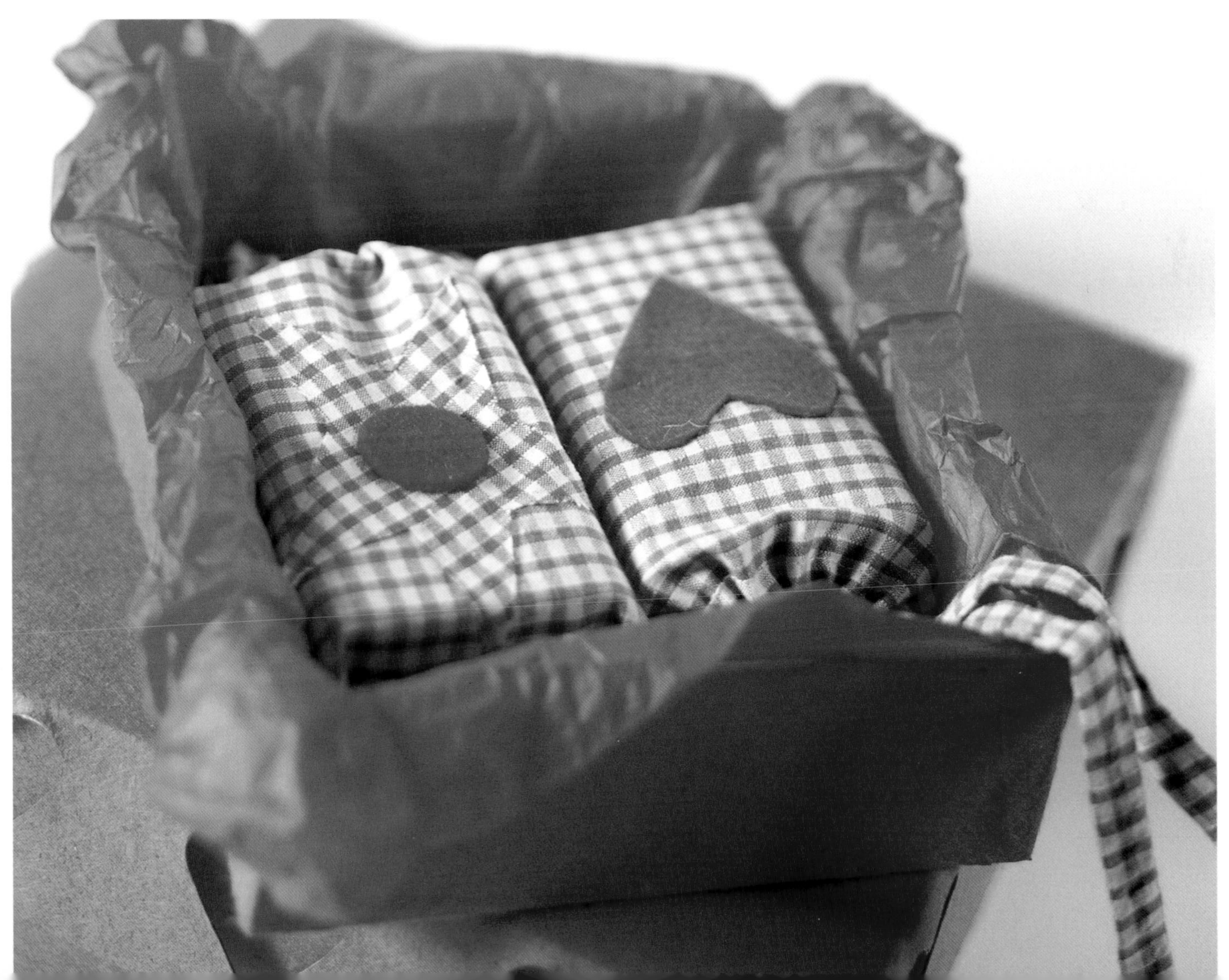

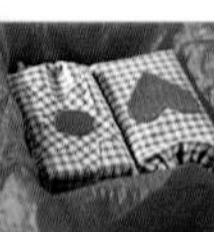

you will need:

blue/white and purple/white gingham fabric

tape measure

scissors

dressmaking pins

iron

sewing machine

white sewing thread

sewing needle

strong fabric glue

piece of card

large-eyed needle

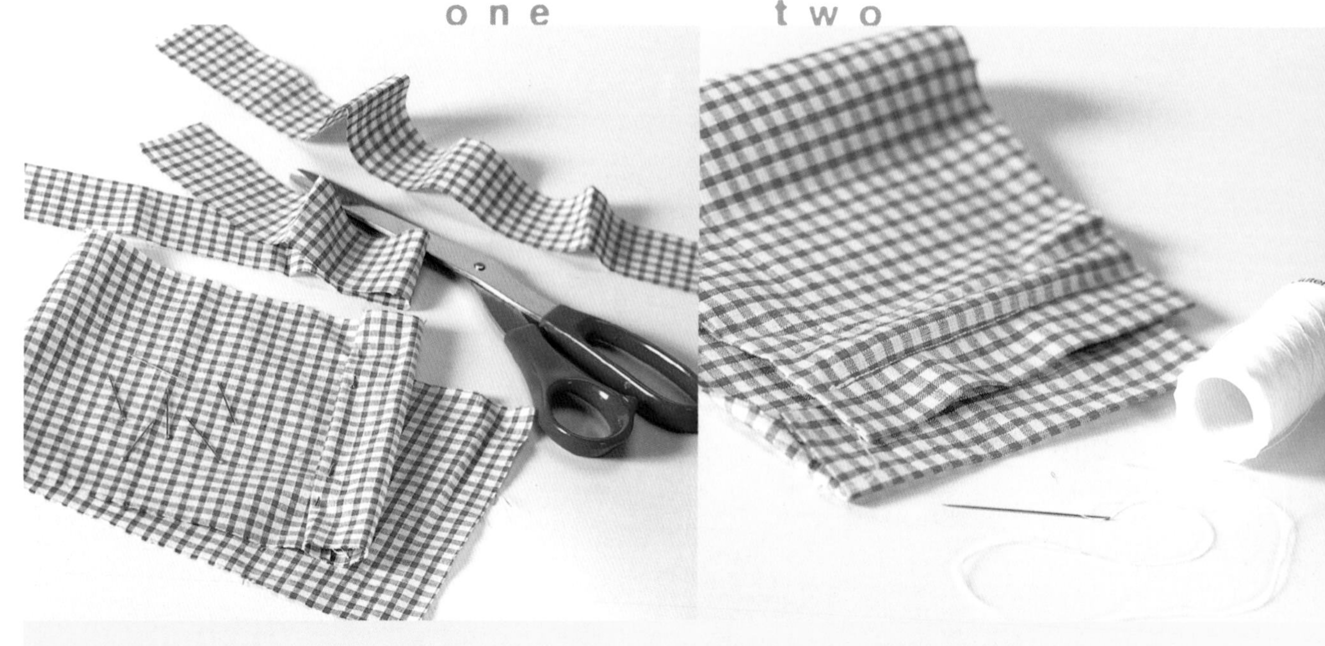

step 1 Cut a rectangle of blue/white gingham 16 inches long and 4 inches wide. Turn over a 2-inch hem to the wrong side on both short edges. Secure with pins.

step 2 Turn over a small hem on both long edges, making sure that the 2-inch hems are uppermost. Fix in position with an iron. Sew two parallel rows of machine-stitching across the 2-inch turnovers. One line of stitching should be on the edge of the turnover, the second line ¾ inch above. These form the channels for the drawstring.

step 3 Fold the fabric in half lengthways, right sides facing. Machine-stitch up both sides, stopping short of the seams running across the top of the bag. Turn the bag right side out.

Cut a strip of blue/white gingham 12 inches long and 1 inch wide. Fold this in half and fold in the raw edges to form a narrow tube. Slip-stitch the edges together to make the drawstring.

step 4 Cut out stars and heart motifs from the purple/white gingham and the red felt. You can choose other motifs if you like. Glue the motifs to the bag with strong fabric glue. Before gluing, insert a piece of card inside the bag to prevent the glue seeping through.

step 5 Thread the drawstring through the channels using a large-eyed needle. Pull the drawstring tight to close the bag.

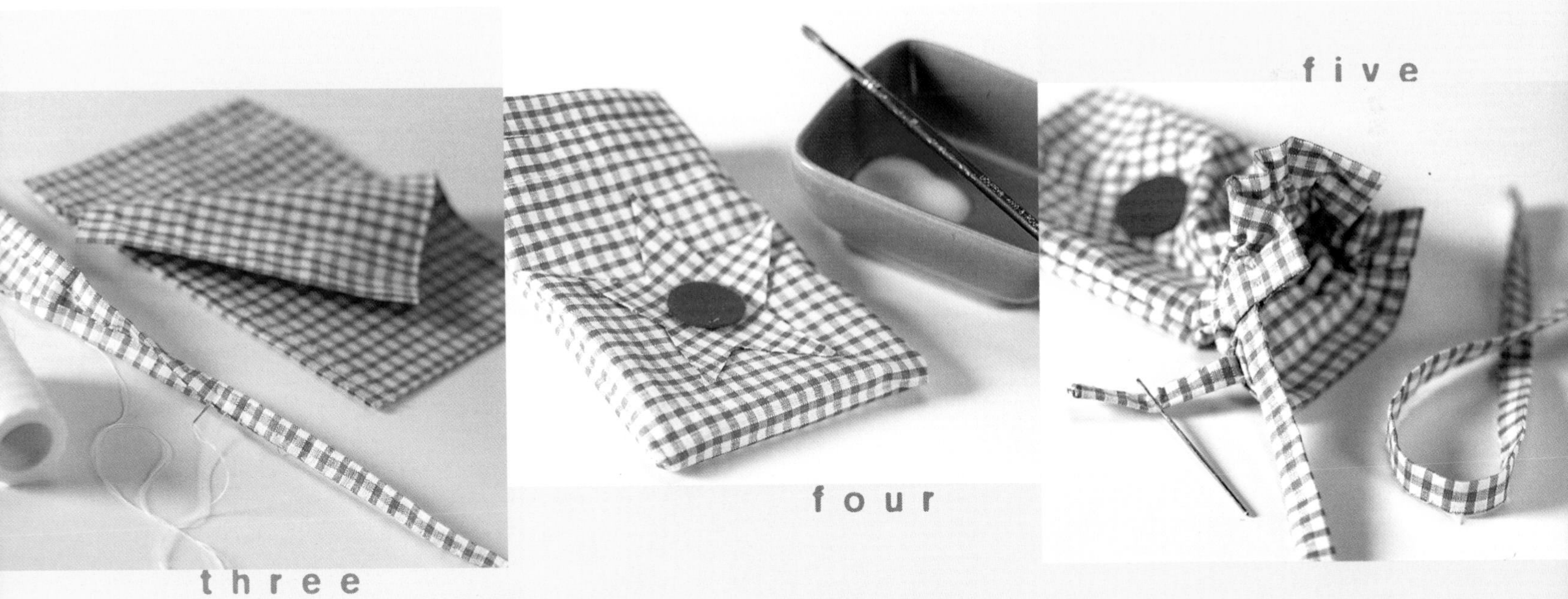

TRADITIONAL ORANGE AND CLOVE POMANDERS

Orange and clove pomanders date back to the seventeenth century when members of the English aristocracy carried pomanders to ward off the Black Death. Nowadays, pomanders are appreciated for their comforting smell and the simple satisfaction of making them.

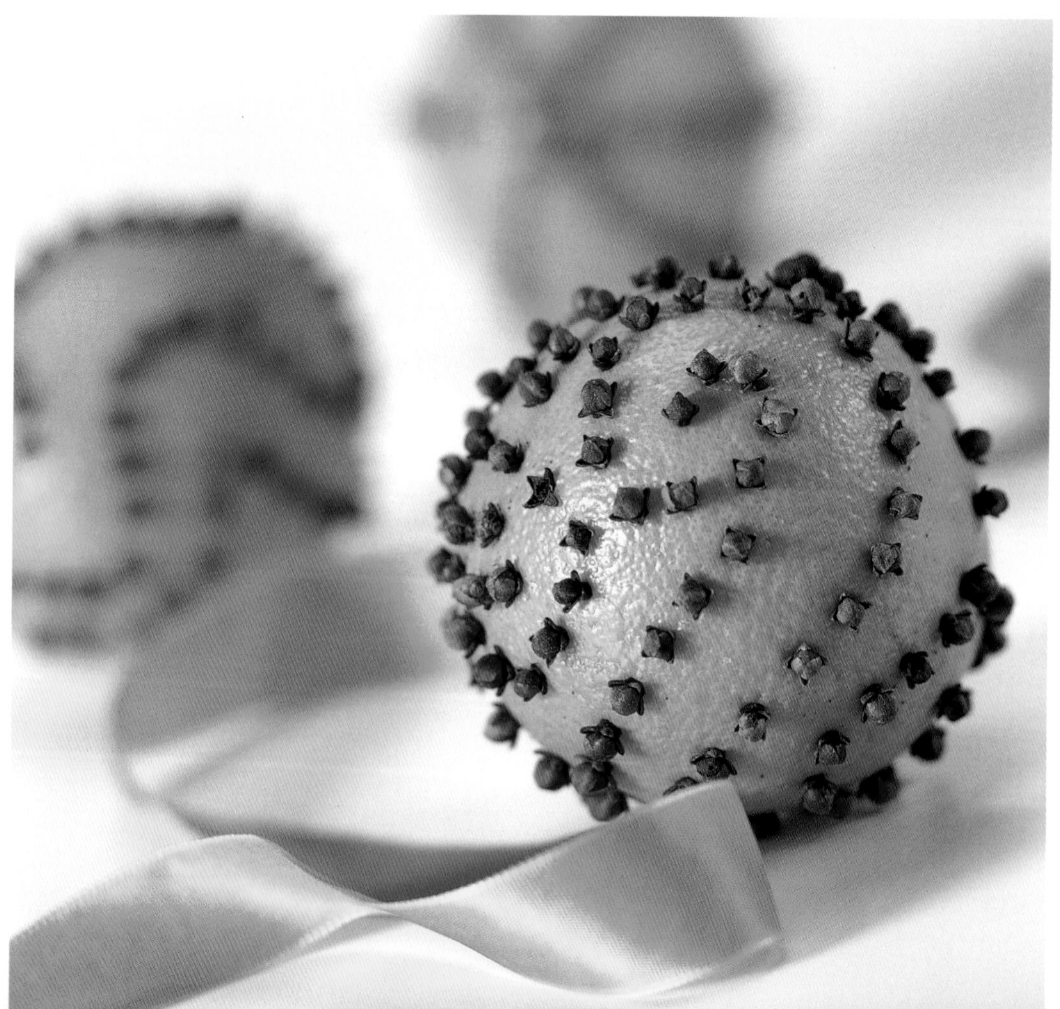

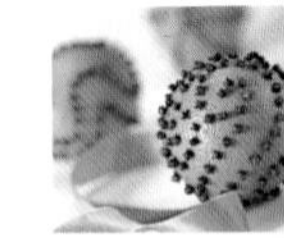

you will need:

1 large orange

fine-tipped marker pen

bradawl

cloves

dried marjoram or Chinese five-spice and ginger spices

one two

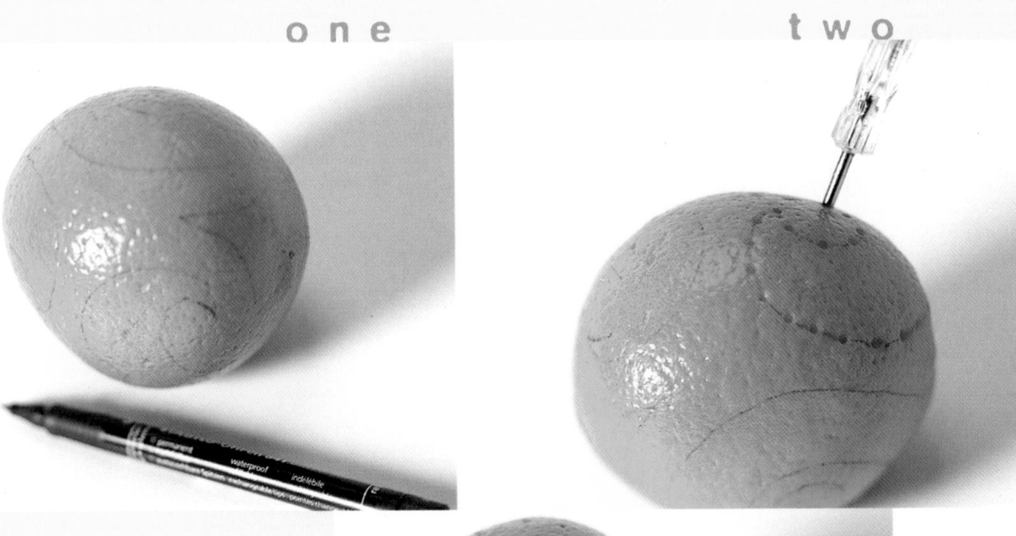

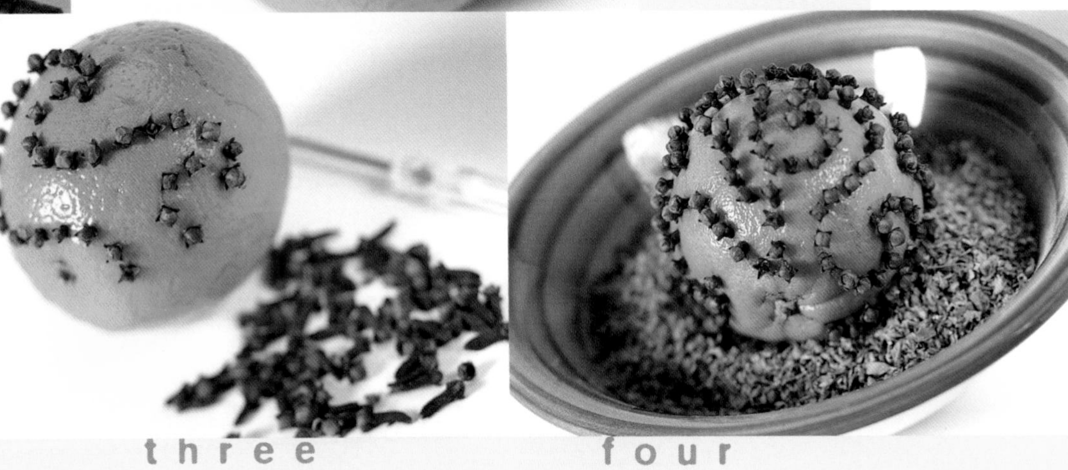

three four

step 1 Using a fine-tipped marker pen, draw a design onto the orange.

step 2 Pierce holes along the lines you have drawn using a bradawl. Leave enough space between each hole to allow for shrinkage, because as the orange dries it will shrivel.

step 3 Push the cloves firmly into each hole as far they will go. The cloves will also shrink as they dry and they may fall out.

step 4 When all the holes have been filled and your design is complete, place the orange in a bowl of herbs or spices. Cover and leave it for 1 to 2 days. Remove the orange from the bowl and leave it in a dark, dry, and warm place for 2 weeks to allow it to dry out.

JEWELED SPICE BALL

This ball is inspired by the Elizabethan pomander but given a contemporary twist with *faux* embellishment. The casing around the twig sphere can be opened so that fresh potpourri, herbs, spices, or essential oils can be added and the fragrance replenished.

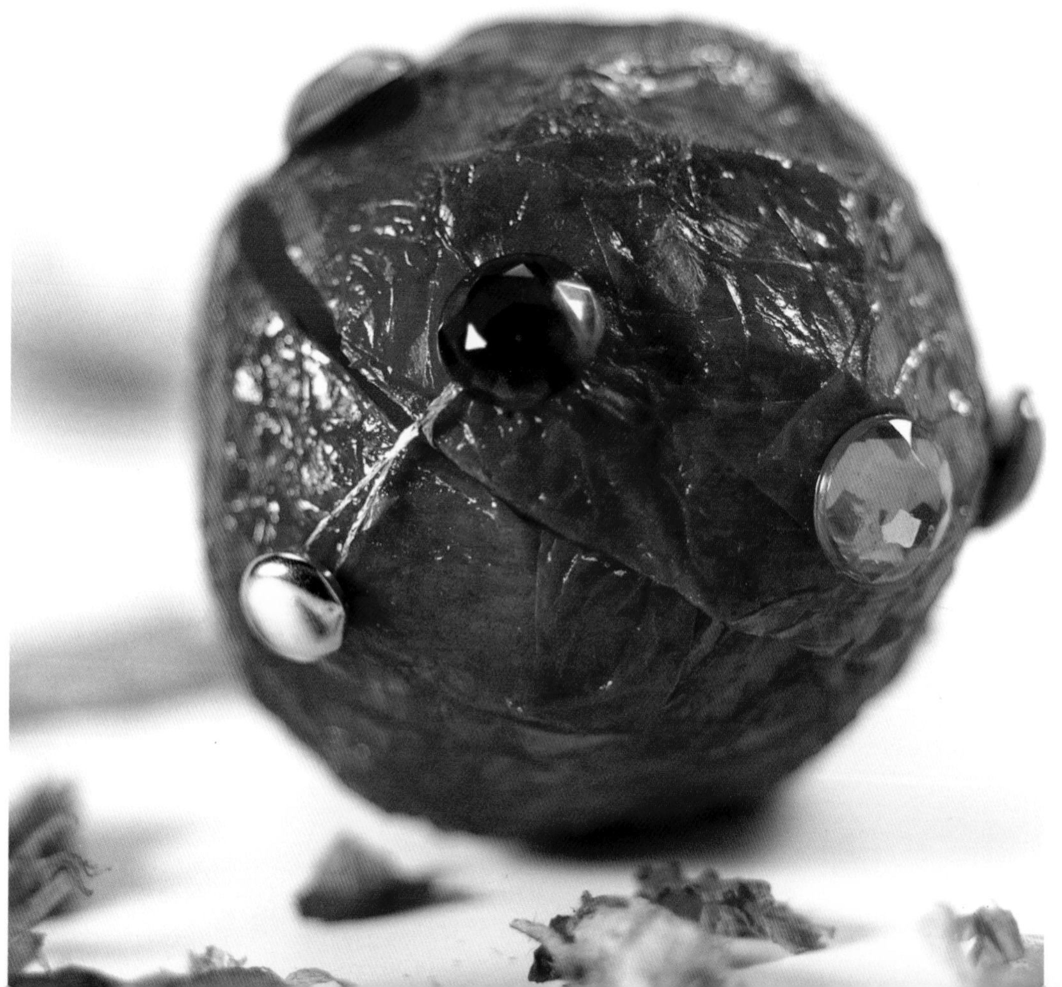

step 1 Cover the rubber ball with layers of plastic food wrap. This will protect the ball and make it easy to remove the papier-mâché. Dampen the tissue paper with a generous amount of glue applied with a brush. Glue the tissue paper around the ball, squeezing it to remove any pockets of air. Allow this layer to dry before continuing.

step 2 Continue adding tissue paper, allowing each layer to dry before applying the next, until you have built up 4 to 5 layers. When the last layer is dry, draw a line all around the ball, making sure that the two halves are equal. Cut along this line with a craft knife.

step 3 Using needle and thread, stitch the two halves together at one point. The stitches will act as a hinge, allowing you to open and close the ball. Make a small hole near the edge of one of the halves, push through a paper binder, and open prongs at back. In a similar position on the other half, use needle and gold thread to sew a loop. The loop must be able to slip over the paper binder.

step 4 Sew another loop at the top of the ball. Attach red and pink glass jewels onto the ball with very strong glue. Position one of the jewels over the loop that connects to the paper binder, as shown. Insert the twig sphere and add your favorite potpourri or a few drops of essential oil. Fasten the ball closed and hang.

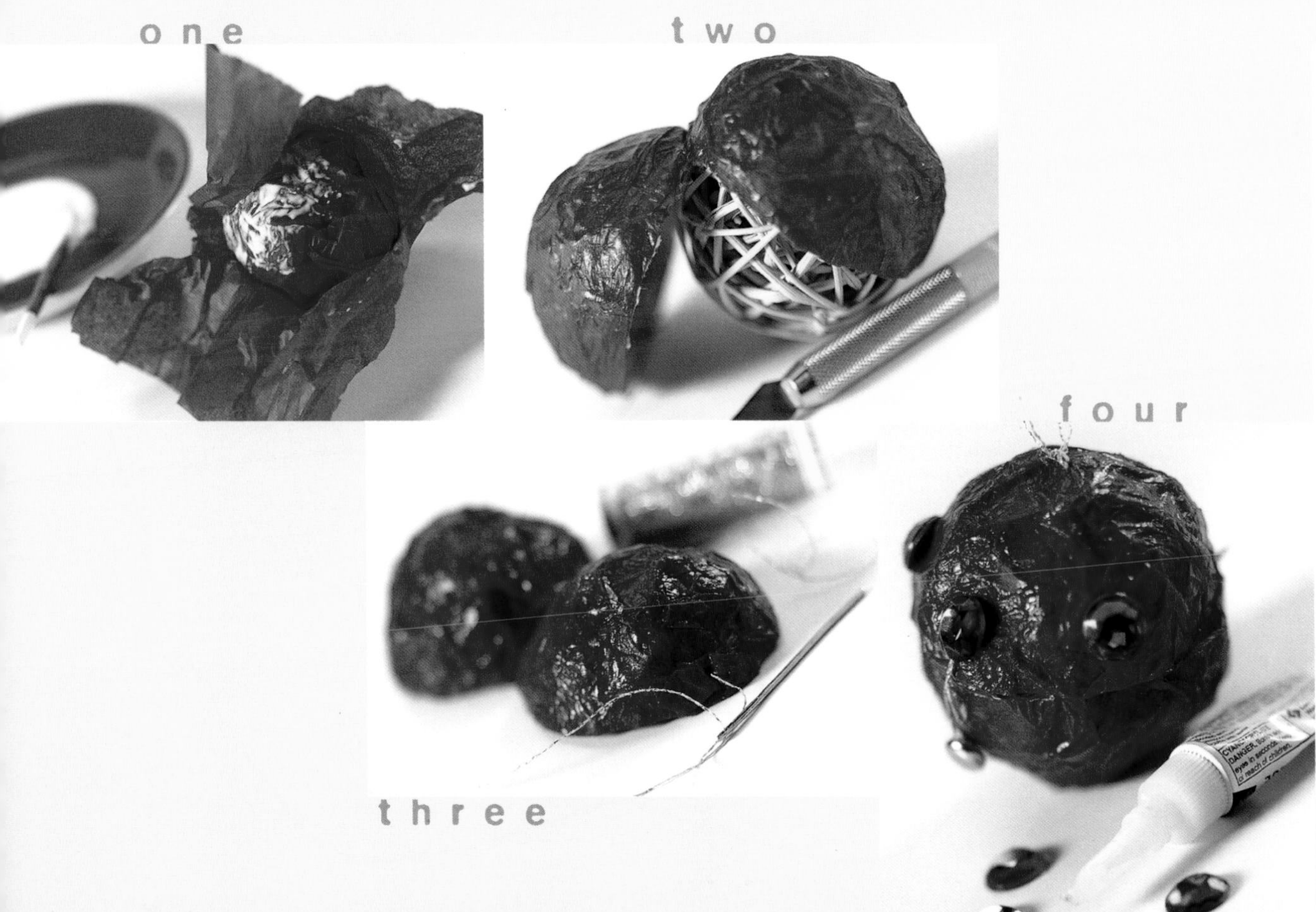

you will need:

rubber ball (slightly larger than the twig sphere)

small twig sphere

plastic food wrap

red tissue paper

strong white glue

brush

pencil

craft knife

sewing needle

gold thread

paper binder

red and pink glass jewels

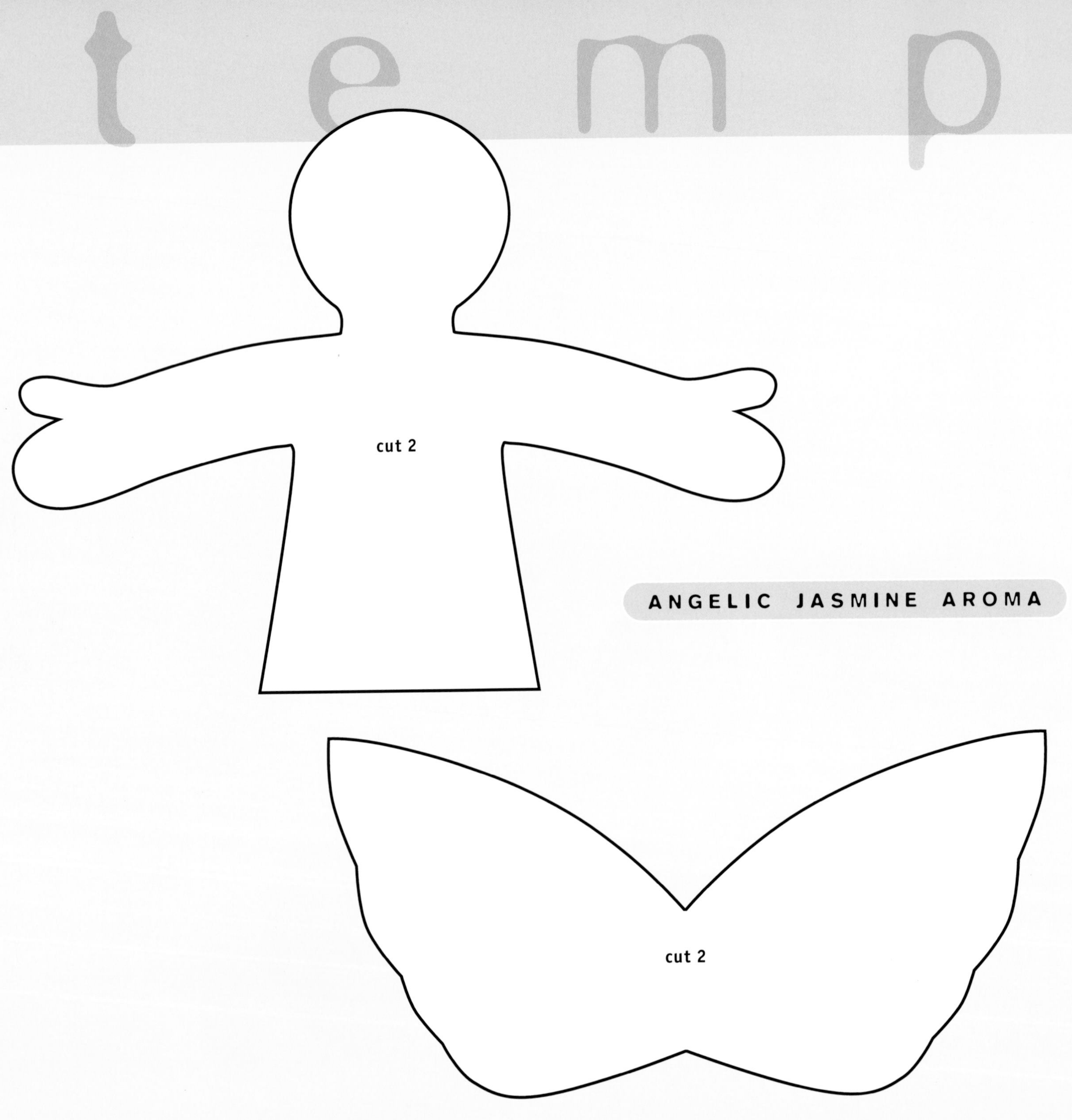
cut 2
ANGELIC JASMINE AROMA
cut 2

EMBOSSED PAPER AND CELESTIAL ESSENTIAL OIL BURNER

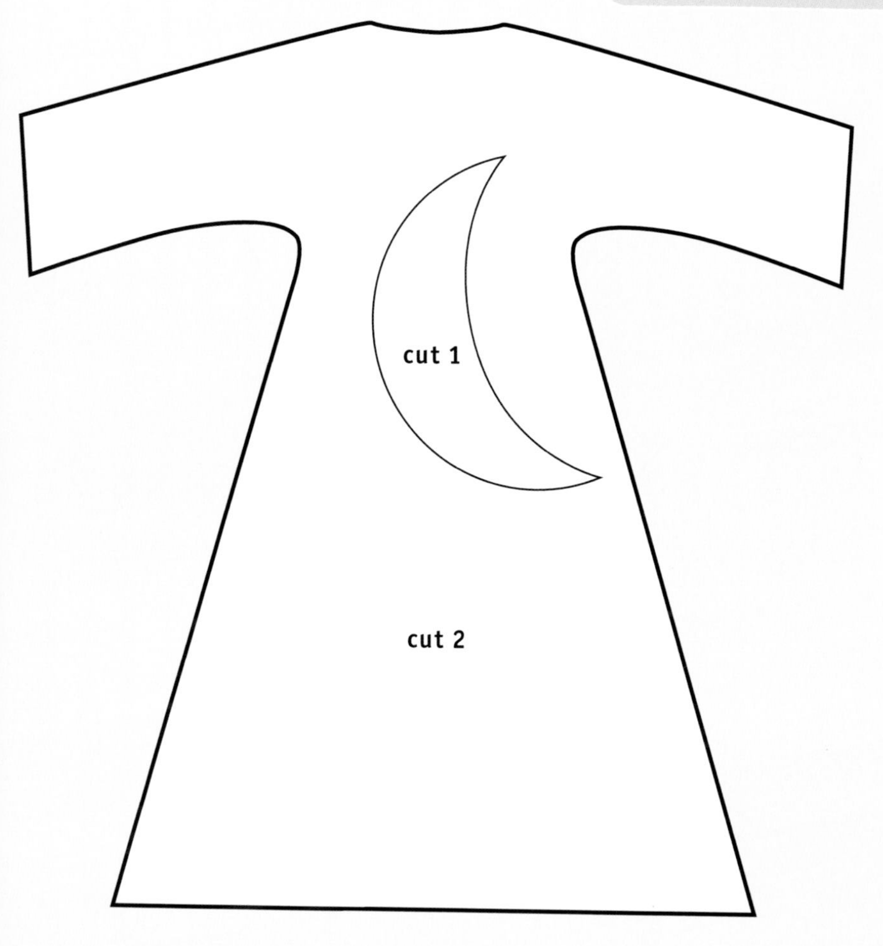

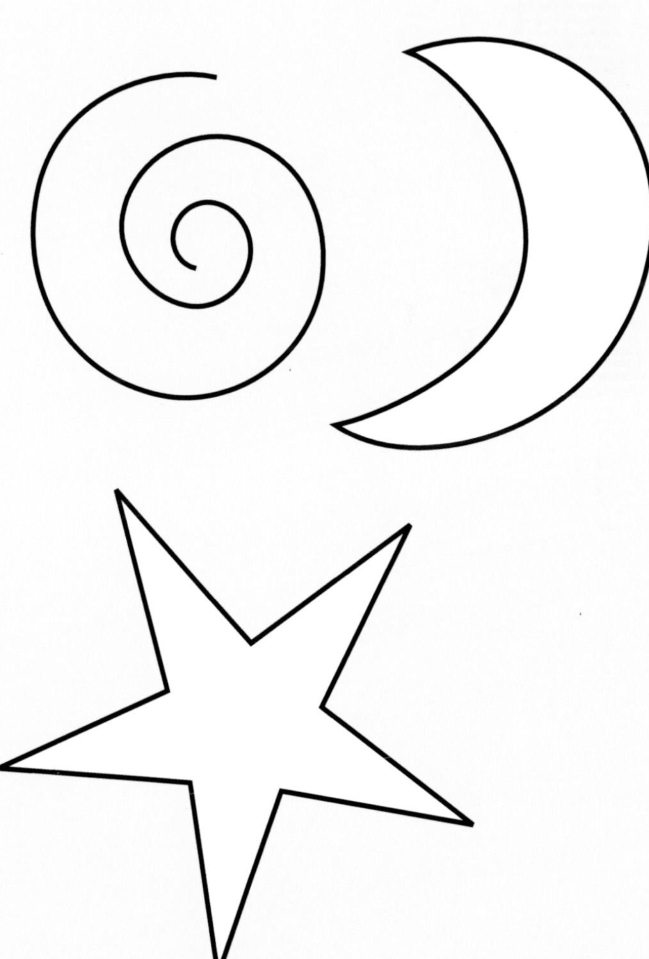

SCENTED ENVELOPES

top flap

envelope I

top flap

envelope II

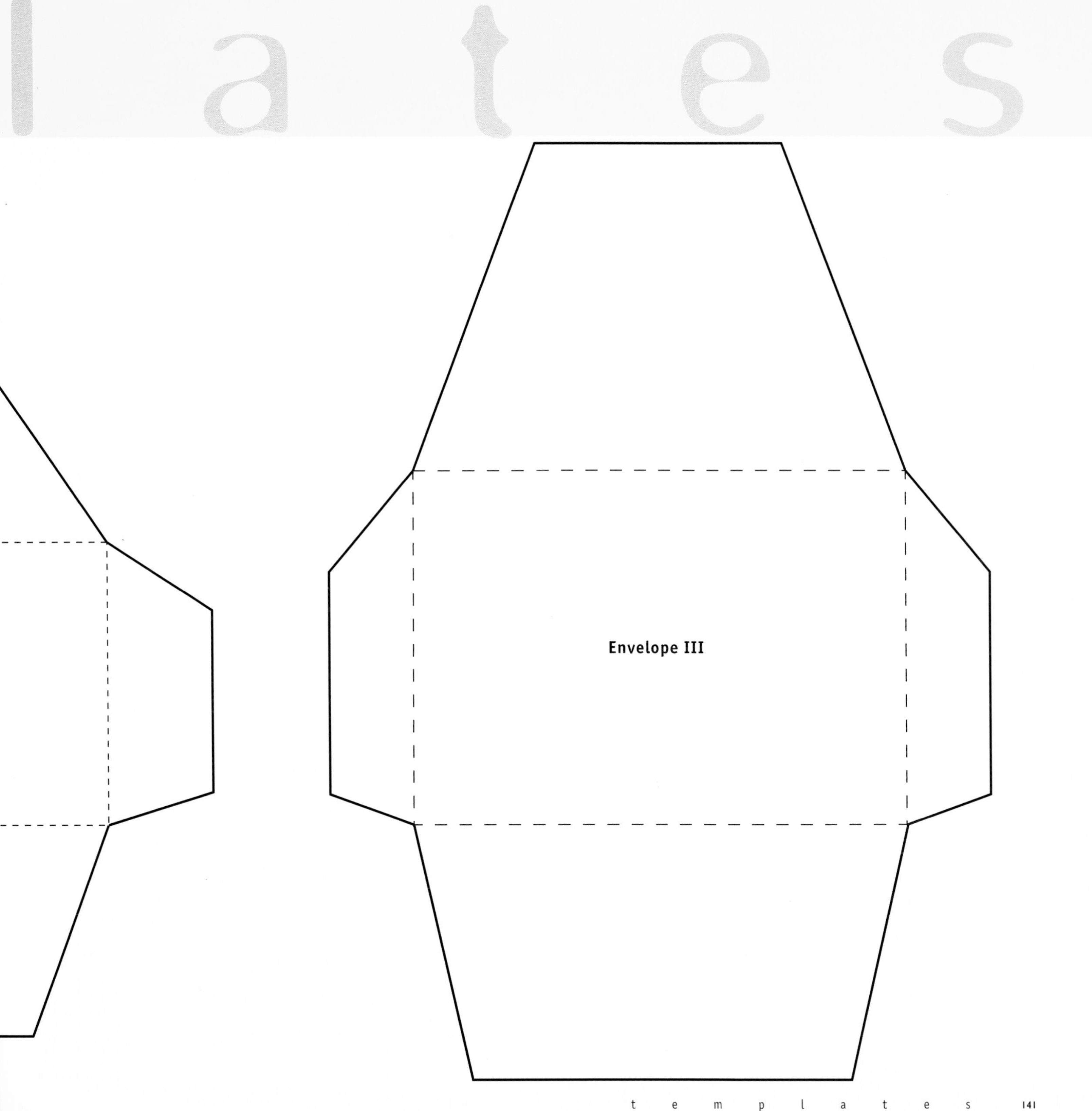
Envelope III

DAISY SACHETS

cut 3 daisies

cut along dotted line

cut 3 centers

cut 1

cut 1

cut 1

MANDARIN-SCENTED TWIG BUNDLES

HEART-SHAPED POTPOURRI BOX AND ROSE-SCENTED HEART SWAG

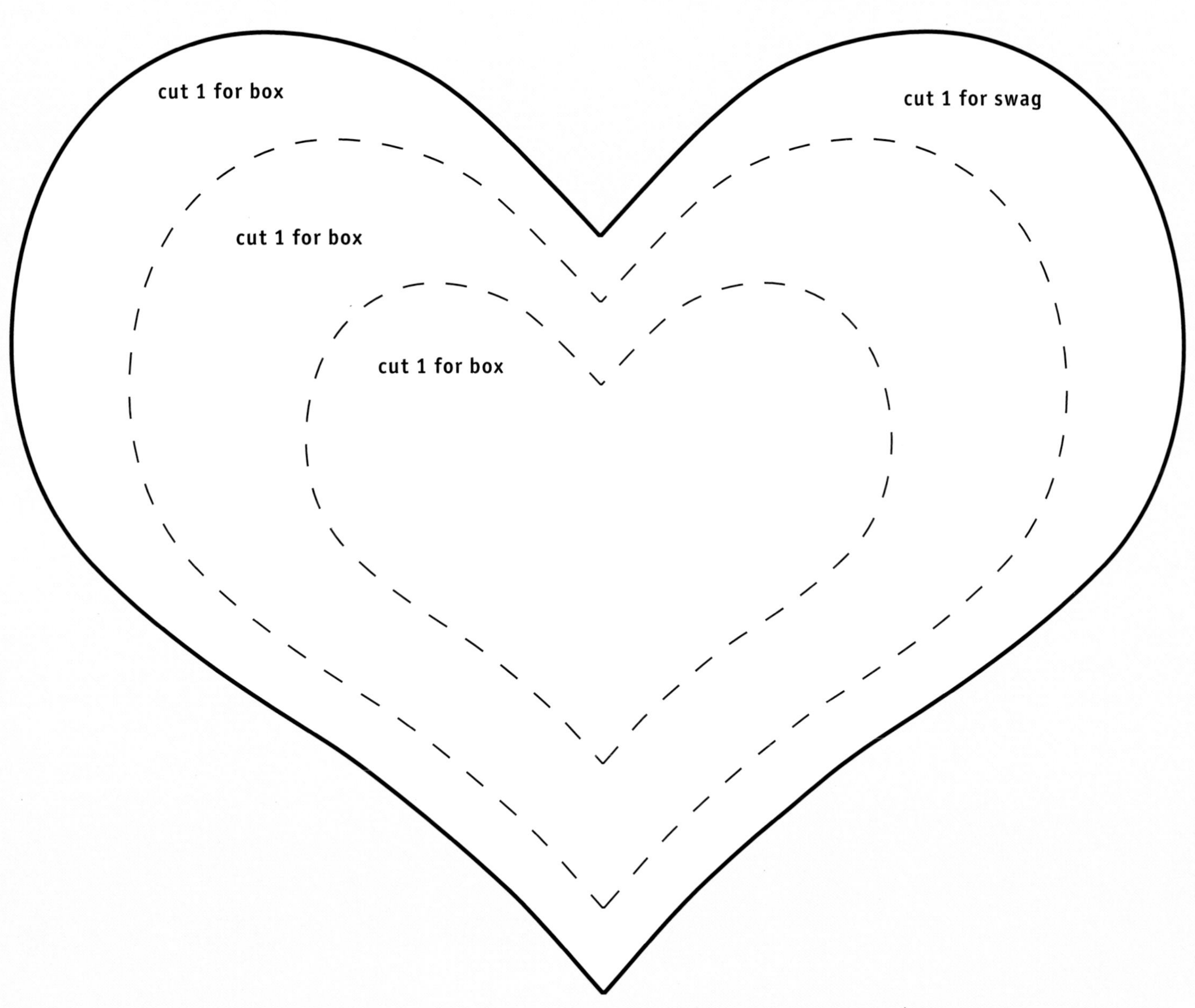

Index

a

ambergris 13
Angel, Scented 54-6
aromatherapy 38-51

b

basil 44
Bath Oils, Scented 96-7
bergamot 44
Body Lotions, Scented 102-3
Book Cover, Chamomile 78-9

c

Carrier Box for Essential Oils 68-9
cedarwood 44
chamomile 44-5
Chamomile Book Cover 78-9
Chamomile Sleep Pillow 94-5
chemical solvents, use of 23
Chile & Rush Paper Greeting Card 77
chocolate 26
Christmas Decorations 118-19
chypre fragrances 28
cinnamon 45
Cinnamon & Bark Paper Greeting Card 77
Cinnamon Candles 114-15
Cinnamon & Gold Mesh Wrapping 58
clove 45
Clove Candles 114-15
clary sage 45
Coat Hangers, Padded Scented 128-30
cold steeping 12

d

Dewberry Sleep Pillow 94-5

e

eau de Cologne 33
eau de parfum 33
eau de toilette 33
Egypt , Ancient 9-10
enfleurage 12,22
Envelopes, Scented 66-7
eucalyptus 45
expression 22
extrait 33

f

Face Cleansing Pack 84-6
Fan, Lavender 126-7
floral fragrances 29-30
fougère fragrances 30
frankincense 46
French perfume making, early 15-17

g

geranium 46
Gift Tags 60-1
Gift Wrapping 57-9
Ginger 46
Grapefruit 47
Greece, Ancient 10-11
Greeting Cards 75-7

h

Hand Cream, Lavender 107-9
Hebrews, Ancient 11

j

jasmine 13,47
juniper 47

l

lavender 47-8
Lavender & Corrugated Cardboard Greeting Card 77
Lavender Cubes 90-1
Lavender Fan 126-7
Lavender Hand Cream 107-9
Lavender Scented Shoe Trees 105-6
lemon balm 48
lemon oil 48
Lemon Soap Balls 87-9
limbic system 8,40
Lip Balm, Vanilla 92-3

m

maceration 12
Mandarin-Scented Twig Bundle 120-1
marine/ocean fragrances 32
marjoram 48
massage 40
melissa 48
mood-altering perfumes 33-4
Mulled Spice Bundles 112-13
musk 13-14
myrrh 48

n

neroli 23

o

oils, essential 38-51
  Burner 122-3
  Carrier Box 68-9
oils, extraction methods 12,22-3
orange blossom 23
orange oil 49
oriental fragrances 30-2
orris 23-4

p

Paper, Embossed 64-5
Paper Roll, Scented 62-3
patchouli 14,49
peppermint 49-50
Peppermint Gift Tags 60-1
Peppermint & Papyrus Greeting Card 76
Perfume Pouches, Velvet 80-1
pine oil 50
pomanders 17
Pomanders, Traditional Orange & Clove 134-5
Potpourri, Rose 98-9
Potpourri Box 72-4
Potpourri Posies 59
pressing 12

r

Romans, Ancient 11-12
room fragrances 41
rose oil 24,50
Rose Potpourri 98-9
Rose & Sandalwood Cleansing Face Pack 84-6
Rose-Scented Heart Swag 116-17
Rosebud Topiary Tree 124-5
rosemary 50
rosewater 14
Rosewater Tonic 100-1

s

Sachets, Daisy 70-1
saffron 14
sandalwood 14-15
Sandalwood & Rose Cleansing Face Pack 84-6
Shoe trees, Lavender-Scented 104-6
Sleep Pillow 94-5
Soap Bag, Gingham 131-3
Soap Balls , Lemon 87-9
Spice Ball, Jeweled 136-7
spikenard 15
steam distillation 22-3
synthetic essences 24-5

t

tea tree 51
Tonic, Rosewater 100-1
Tree, Rosebud 124-5
Twig Bundle, Mandarin-Scented 120-1

v

vanilla 24
Vanilla-Scented Lip Balm 92-3

y

ylang-ylang 24,51

Picture Credits

Heather Angel: pages 22 (right), 23, 24; Archive Photos France: pages 8, 19; e.t. archive: pages 9, 10 (left), 11, 16, 18: Papilio Photographic: page 22 (left); Courtesy Jean Patou: page 26; Rochas: pages 32, 35 (right), and Roger Viollet: pages 10 (right), 13, 14, 15.